DISCOVER EXER-SEX.

Your Love Life Will Never Be The Same.

No matter how many sex manuals you read or different methods you try, you will probably never experience the *total* joy of sex until your body is healthy and fit.

Noted physical fitness expert Bonnie Prudden wrote *EXER-SEX* to show you that possessing an attractive, flexible, strong, well-trained body is not a matter of luck or inheritance: good lovers are made, not born. Crammed with amusing anecdotes, sound advice and dozens of fabulous, fun-to-follow *sexercises* to help you slim down and shape up, *EXER-SEX* shows that anyone can have a rich, exciting, satisfying love life. You can too.

ABOUT THE AUTHOR

Bonnie Prudden has been a world -class authority on physical fitness and exercise since the 1950s. Her research on the fitness of American children led to the formation of the President's council on Physical Fitness during the Eisenhower administration. Her innovations include the first pre and postnatal exercise programs, the first baby exercise program, the first swim program designed especially for infants, and the first exercise program designed for older people. At various times Ms. Prudden has contributed to a regular column in *Sports Illustrated*, held a regular spot on *"The Today Show"* and set up scores of programs in schools, YM & YWCAs, camps, prisons, and recreation centers throughout the country. She has been inducted into the Physical Fitness Hall of Fame, the Massage Hall of Fame and is the recipient of the President's Council Lifetime Achievement Award. She is the director of Bonnie Prudden Myotherapy, Inc. in Tucson, Arizona.

www.bonnieprudden.com

BONNIE PRUDDEN BOOKS

Pain Erasure the Bonnie Prudden Way
Myotherapy: Bonnie Prudden's Complete Guide to Pain-Free Living
Bonnie Prudden's After Fifty Fitness Guide
Your Baby Can Swim
How to Keep Your Child Fit From Birth to Six
Teenage Fitness
How to Keep Your Family Fit and Healthy
How to Keep Slender and Fit After Thirty
Exer-Sex

EXER-SEX

Exercises for Sex, for Love, for Life

BY BONNIE PRUDDEN

Illustrated by James Dubbs

**Everyone we ever love teaches us . . .
This book is dedicated most gratefully
to those whom *I* have loved.**

EXER-SEX: EXERCISES FOR SEX,
FOR LOVE, FOR LIFE

ISBN: 1-4663-7855-7
ISBN-13: 9781466378551

Contents

Foreword

Oh, dear! All those lovely books on sex, lavishly illustrated in living color, telling you exactly how to do it. ("Insert tab A into slot B," et cetera, et cetera.) Everyone telling you how to, but nobody telling you what with.

The assumption is that the mere possession of a body and a bit of know-how ensures one a life of endless sexual joy. Not so! That's like taking a neophyte of average physique, handing him a book of instructions, taking him to the top of a steep ski slope, equipping him with boots, ski poles, and skis, and then shoving him down the hill. His chances of failure, without preliminary exercises to strengthen his ankles and improve his flexibility and bodily skills, would be quite impressive.

If you want to become an expert skier, you must develop your body into an instrument for skiing. And if you want to become an expert lovemaker you must develop your body into an instrument for making love. Possessing an attractive, flexible, strong, well-trained body is not a matter of luck or inheritance. Good lovers are self-made, not born. You'd be surprised at the degree of control you have over your body, including your looks.

As for the "sexercises" themselves, the very names of many of the exercises I am going to teach you in this book demonstrate their function in making you a more skillful and adept lover: the pelvic tilt, the hip swing, the circle tilt, the crotch stretch. Most of these exercises are ecumenical, equally beneficial to men and women, but where they are intended for one sex only, I'll let you know.

Remember, when you possess a wonderful instrument, you are more apt to use it, and you certainly take—and give—more pleasure in its use. This book is devoted to helping you—with a little sweat of your brow in the process—turn your body into such an instrument.

Let's keep in mind, however, that the act of love is more than physical. That's only one side of the triangle, though a very important one. The other two are the mental and the spiritual sides. Cultivate all three and you will have an enviable love life.

In the first chapter I am going to talk to you about sexuality and nonverbal, body-to-body communication. In the second chapter I am going to talk about how the way you think can affect the way you move—and a few other things. And *then* we'll get down to cases and I will show you how to develop certain muscles and control certain motions so that your body becomes an instrument of greater pleasure for you and your partner than you ever dreamed possible.

1

It's Not All in Your Head . . . Thank God!

Communication with others is the only defense we have against the hardest thing man has to bear, loneliness; and the first instance of communication for each of us is sexual.

At a certain time in our life span, a cataclysm occurs in darkness and in silence. A part of what we are to become penetrates deep into a second, and the two become one. We are born only because one body communicated sexually with another, and because the first two parts of ourselves met and communicated sexually. We then spend the first months of our growing deep in sexual territory, often sharing, by virtue of proximity and chemical dependence, in the sexual unions of those to whom we owe our existence. When we finally emerge, protesting the pain and indignity of our forced ejection from that secret place so well-fitted to our needs, we leave through a sexual portal. All the rest of our lives we will relate sexually to everyone else, even when we are totally unaware of it. From this second on, however, *you* will never be totally unaware again. Since this is a fact, perhaps it would be well to have a clear idea of what sexuality really is.

Sexuality is not to be confused with the word "sex." The word "sex" is a short, blunt word, sometimes used to denote whether a person is male or female. Of late, it has come to mean much more—and at the same time much less. It falls far short of describing the precious quality we all possess—sexuality. The word "sex" means different things to each of us; sexuality is the same for all.

All during those months *in utero,* as we put ourselves together, we are prepared for the best that sexuality has to offer. Our skin, so new, so sensitive, and so *alive,* is held close-pressed against a smooth wall. As we move, the warm enveloping sides slide against our backs, buttocks, crowns, shoulders, arms, legs, and even the soles of our feet. Warm water surrounds and cushions us against sudden movement even as it rocks us. It filters disturbing sounds but it amplifies the primitive drumbeat of the great heart that supplies everything required for life.

Lines of communication within us begin the second *we* begin, and they soon spread into a network of electric conduits, relays, and programmed computers. We have ample proof of this when we step on a thorn that flashes "stepped on something sharp," or when we touch a hot stove. In that instance the computers even bypass central intelligence and go into emergency action before there is time consciously to assess the danger. Split seconds before we get the message "touched hot stove," the endangered hand has been removed and is being waved briskly in cooling air. We also set up lines of communication with that intelligence that is in our immediate vicinity—mother—but instead of using connecting lines, we use something that might be called ESP. Wise is the woman who speaks loving, comforting, encouraging, *welcoming* words to the child within.

Nonverbal communication is also a fact of life. It seems reasonable to expect it between a mother and her unborn child, but there is ample evidence pointing to communication taking place even before life, as we know it, takes place—with ova that have not even been fertilized.

Hen's eggs are also ova. The ones you buy in the store are usually infertile; the average hen in America never gets even close to a rooster. Yet when hen's eggs are broken, which means being destroyed as far as the egg is concerned, they are able to communicate that fact to plants wired to polygraphs. And the polygraphs in turn are able to communicate that destruction to man. With these phenomena in mind, we would be foolish to think of our own beginnings as lacking either sensation or the means to communicate with *someone.*

Old wives (who, it seems, were often wiser than we thought) had it that "shock would mark the child." Science, which once laughed indulgently at this ancient pronouncement, now says that, yes, shocks that activate the adrenals and other powerful hormones could indeed affect a growing fetus. What neither the old wives nor modern science has mentioned, but what most *healthy,* sensitive women know instinctively, is that they can communicate with their unborn babies. Sometimes they do it with thought, and sometimes with words. Whatever the method of sending and receiving, the two are on the same wavelength, and just because you cannot see a radio wave is no proof that it does not exist. What comes across to the unborn is a *feeling* of love, and love cannot be divorced from sexuality. Such children are also "marked"—but with contentment, with a sense of security and love.

Birth is a painful, terrifying process from which some of us never recover, and our very first rewards for having survived the experience are sexual. We are held tenderly in hands that are alive and that *communicate.* There is no such thing as touching another person without communicating *something.*

Those hands bathe us gently in water that is almost the same temperature as the tiny sea that has just cast us up on an alien shore. Comforting arms enfold us, patting and rubbing our backs, buttocks, and shoulders. Our heads are supported by communicating fingers.

We are given the breast, an important part of the sexual arsenal that will confront us all the rest of our days. Through it comes the life that once coursed into us from the drumming heart, which can be heard again, even though from a distance. As we suck that life into ourselves, we cause impulses to flow along nerves that carry them straight to the uterus we have so recently left. The effect is to stimulate it to contract, and to contract again and again, soon to resume its prenatal size and condition. The effect is rehabilitating. The sensation, however, is sexual.

At birth we don't see very much with our eyes, but we feel with every centimeter of skin. We have no vocabulary but we are capable of voicing our needs to anyone who will listen. We understand no language, yet we know from voice timbre and from *nonverbal communication* what the speaker means and the total context of each message. As we grow older, unless we are actually taught to listen to something that has no name and to feel that same nameless something, we lose the ability to understand. We transfer our attention instead to words, and words have as many meanings as there are people involved in a conversation. If you wish to renew that very special skill you once had, start listening to people with your eyes closed, not closed so you can escape into fantasy, but closed so you can listen via the pathways of *nonverbal communication*.

It isn't just our skin that relays feel. We are also born with a well-developed sense of dynamics. We know full well whether the hands that hold us are sure, experienced, and safe, or something else. This fact has embarrassed more than one unsuspecting mother who has had to repossess a screaming baby from the arms of a doting (potentially smothering or secretly rejecting) relative. Facial expression, smiles, and honeyed words carry no weight at all with babies; they get all their information straight from the sender with no chance of a foul-up at a relay station. They will have it long enough (for about eighteen months) to lay down the entire foundation for their lives. By the time this sense starts to fade and the open circuits close, one by one, their computers will be loaded with information that will never be totally erased. Hopefully, they will begin their lives (from the moment of conception) surrounded by love. Later on in life we all get confused about love, with love, and by love, but not babies. They have the facts.

The first months of our lives are filled with sexuality in the best sense of the word. It is more stimulating and fulfilling than it will ever be again—sex education, sex advertisements, sex images, sex games, sex literature, and sex freedom to the contrary. As babies, our skin is bathed daily by a willing and loving slave. Our sensitive skin answers totally to enveloping hands, more completely than it ever will in the years to come. Oh, that won't be because we will never be quite so sensitive again. Eventually, most of our sexual sensitivity will center in areas we call erogenous; as babies, we are totally erogenous.

When you are a baby, your brand-new button nose, unscarred by the acids of pollution, smells everything. Your first association with skin and its special perfume is tied to caresses, comfort, and food. It should not be surprising then that, one day, eating will be tied to sexuality, either as a prelude to lovemaking or, alas, instead of. Caresses, bodily comfort, nourishment, and pleasant odors all have sexual undertones.

In the beginning, sexuality is purely physical, but it soon develops many facets that will be dependent on the mind, personality, character, experience, self-image, state of health, and intensity of drive of each person. It is further dependent on the chance that engineers our meetings with others. In recent years many books have been written on the subject of sex, most of them "how-to" manuals dealing with mechanics. When you are reading these books, try to keep in mind that "how to" is the least important part of lovemaking. What is very important, in fact indispensable, is the understanding not of *sex* but of *sexuality*. Rather than try to remember seventy-five positions, try to retain your gift of sexuality, a gift that didn't come to you with puberty but at conception—when you were tender, sensitive, and open for nonverbal communication. When you can do that, then "how to" serves a purpose.

2

Fit for Sex, Anyone?

The summer I was ten and at Camp Manhansack on Shelter Island, one of my bunkmates called a meeting under the Arts and Crafts Building. She had chosen three of us for her lecture, and we waited expectantly as she warmed up the audience with dire threats as to what she would do if we told *anyone*. Then she explained where babies came from *and how they got there in the first place.* My immediate reaction was, "Oh you made that up!" Her scornful, "You'll see!" followed me as I stumped indignantly upstairs to the rec room with its less exotic chatter.

As soon as I got home from camp I told my mother I'd heard something strange at camp, something about where babies came from *and how they got there in the first place* . . . and was it true? My mother was too wary to get caught on that one, so she said, "You tell me what you heard and I'll tell you if it's true." So I did, with all the color and exactitude afforded by my ten-year-old vocabulary (very different from the one in vogue with today's young) and my informant's somewhat limited knowledge concerning male and female anatomy. "Essentially that's correct," said my mother. Later I learned that my information was *essentially* incorrect, but that *geographically* I had it right. My mother then added that I was not to tell my friends anything of what we had discussed, since mothers preferred to be the ones to impart such important information to their children. It was four years before I began to wonder when my mother intended to impart the whole of it to me. She never did.

In those days sex was something most people thought about a great deal but discussed only in the most indirect terms. For some it was wonderful, for others repetitious and dull. A few wished it had never been invented. Most children found out about it as I did, under the Arts and Crafts Building, in the cloakroom, behind the barn, or just walking home from school with older children. The startling news fell onto ground well-prepared by ignorance and inhibition. It was then cultivated and fertilized with misinformation. Such books as were then available to the average individual were usually entitled *How to Have a Happy Marriage* and seemed to have been written by perennially menopausal people whose most intimate relationships must have been with the *Encyclopaedia Britannica.* Was it any wonder Freud was listened to with avidity when he let sex out of the trunk? Anything that bore any relationship at all to truth was infinitely preferable to the fantasy dished out by everyone from parent to pastor. The pendulum commenced to swing—swing, swang, swung—and now where are we?

Inhibitions are a thing of the past, and if you admit to any, you are supposedly not quite all right. Ignorance too is gone. My grandson didn't have to wait to be ten and go to camp to get his facts. He was four when he gave me all the details, both essential and geographical, of his baby brother's conception, womb life, and birth. The facts were both extensive and correct. And who was startled? His grandmother. Now just about everyone, no matter how young, is aware of sex both subconsciously and consciously; it's impossible to miss it. Today the number engaged in it in any one place and time depends on the leanings of those involved. All the old hang-ups have been exposed, and in this sexually aware age everything should be almost perfect. Why is it, then, that some folks find sex wonderful, some think it dull and repetitious, and some wish it had never been invented? Is it possible that some factor other than the twin dreadfuls, ignorance and inhibition, is at work? Without question there is such a factor—and that factor is *a low level of sexuality.*

Today the *How to Have a Happy Marriage* books have been shouldered aside by a host of "how-to" manuals so replete with illustrations and step-by-step instructional procedures that every youngster over the age of nine knows "how to," even though the equipment is still in the developmental stage. The tragedy that stalks this enlightened generation is caused by neither ignorance concerning sex nor inhibition. It is caused by a new way of life, and this new way of life has robbed millions of the "with what" to "how to."

Sex begins in your head, but it doesn't stay there. At its best, it is a physical expression, a symbol of the need to give and to receive love. But as a *physical* expression it requires a *physical* body for its consummation, and before it can consummate, it must first desire and then attract. To be sexually attractive, one must also be healthy, and health does not mean the mere absence of an observable ailment. It means being so alive with vibrant *positive* health that it can be seen *and felt* by everyone. More than half the people you pass in the street, sit next to in restaurants, travel with on buses and planes, work with in classrooms, offices, and factories, are not truly healthy, even if they aren't "ill." As a result, they generally aren't attractive, and a closer look will tell you that they aren't sexually attractive either.

A man once told me that every time he entered a crowded room he looked everyone over and asked himself which of the women he would enjoy sleeping with and which of the men he could beat in a fight. Had he chosen to follow either path, his chances of success were excellent. He was a very sexually attractive man, which was immediately apparent to most of the women present. He was also extremely strong and healthy. Using those two questions the next time you enter a room full of people, you will discover something very disconcerting. The selection for sexual activity will be very limited; in fact, the chances are that you won't find one person you would even consider.

On the other hand, if you are healthy yourself, your success on the war front would be almost certainly assured.

There is some weight to the argument that what one person finds sexually attractive might be abhorrent to another, but there are some basic criteria that seem to be universal. See if they are part of your standards for others and ask yourself how *you* stack up. Madison Avenue has spent millions of dollars compiling lists of just such basic attributes of sexuality for a very basic (and, to them, attractive) reason. Such research has been instrumental in parting you and millions like you from your dollars. Advertisers have discovered that if they can catch your attention they have one finger in your wallet. And they know that the best way to do that is to present a very attractive person of either sex using their products. Consciously, you the potential consumer react positively to the attractive person. Subconsciously, you register the brand of cigarette, beer, antiperspirant, bra, or hair dressing which that attractive person is using. The next time you go shopping, you are very likely to spot, and perhaps purchase, that product. Would you have subconsciously registered that particular brand name if you hadn't been made aware of it in connection with something especially pleasing? You would not.

Those millions of Madison Avenue dollars spent on tests to find ways of advertising products that please almost everyone have proven that the advertisement that gets the most immediate and *lasting* response is *sexually pleasing*. They have zeroed in on those outward characteristics that are both powerful and universal in their appeal. What, then, does a sexually pleasing body look like, and how is it used to get the most for the advertiser's dollar? And if it works for Madison Avenue, why not for you?

First examine the setting for the advertisement, because it tells you what the sexually pleasing person seems to do with time. He or she is usually pictured in bright sunlight, at the edge of soaring mountain ranges, walking along a quiet country lane or wooded path, skiing down a sparkling slope, or beneath tall pines. In other words, *attractive people choose to be in action and close to nature.* It is hard to imagine where Madison Avenue could have learned such a thing, but there is tremendous sexuality involved whenever people are free to indulge in nature and in each other.

What about the bodies themselves, whatever the setting? At first glance you will notice that not one of them is ever overweight, not even slightly. It is just not possible to be sexually attractive and fat—not any more than it is possible to be fat and really healthy.

Next, the skin. It is smooth and usually tan. This is meant to reinforce your feeling that these people are connected with fresh air, action, and all outdoors. It also suggests freedom from dull, routine work, and it subtly suggests playtime. The sun plays a particularly active part in advertisements, just as it should play an active part in our lives—but for several reasons may not. The first is because we forget that for all growing things the sun means life, well-being, and even a feeling of contentment and happiness. Moonlight may filter down on scenes of sexual consummation, but if a half-aware exchange has been going on all day as two people lie, play, or even work in the sun, then moonlight has the cooperation of two bodies fully prepared and ready for loving. Compare the way you might feel toward your love after a day spent sailing, hiking, swimming, or just lazing out of doors, with what you might feel after an afternoon of bridge or TV. True, not every day can be spent in activities outdoors, but ask yourself when you last did any of those things . . . and how often you did any of them last year.

Another reason we don't get the most and best from the sun, even if we are wise enough to seek it out, is new to the world. There is so much pollution in the air that many of the sun's valuable rays are filtered out. One doesn't notice pollution while lying next to the pool in the heart of midtown, but go out from the city and look back. That dark yellow haze is filth, and not only does it hang between you and the disc of life, it is riding into and out of your lungs like the rise and fall of a dirty tide. And, yes, constant exposure to pollution does affect sex.

Even when Madison Avenue's hucksters are not advertising products guaranteed to make hair shine, eyes sparkle, skin free of blemish, and teeth white, theirs are. It is well known to hairdressers that when a woman or a man comes into the shop with a picture of a certain style taken from a magazine, asking that his or her own locks be so arranged, the stylist is in trouble. The customer rarely looks at style alone but includes the face beneath it. The model's face and the customer's face may be very different indeed, but the magic has been worked. The handsome or lovely features have been observed, and somehow, if only through desire, assumed.

The magic just described becomes black magic when a model with his rugged, wind-burned features and lean body sitting tall in the saddle whips out a cigarette and lights up. He is the very personification of attractive masculine sexuality. He is also strong and *healthy*. You are consciously aware of his features and posture, you are unconsciously aware that if the smoke he is pulling past those shining teeth and down into what must be healthy lungs doesn't harm *him*, it certainly isn't going to harm *you*. You do the expected, the planned and paid-for. You tie the healthy, attractive model to the product in the totally unfounded belief that you will not only be ruggedly masculine-looking as you light up, but subtly sexy and quite safe from harm. No one even whispers the truth, that smoking is a particularly virulent form of pollution and will most assuredly affect your sex life.

So, the sexually attractive person equates with the healthy attractive person as far as outward appearance goes. What's next?

The Way You Move Speaks Volumes

Madison Avenue, when it applies its arts to television, chooses people who have excellent posture and who move well. Why? Because we are all adept at sizing up people from our very first contact with them, which is usually eye-to-body. In one quick look we can absorb an incredible amount of information. Male; female; tall; short (almost to the inch); weight (almost to the pound); skin color; hair color, style, and texture; body type; posture; clothing; background; and even projected attitude toward the others in the room. At the next party where you meet strangers, take in as much as you can about each one. Later, when you go over your inventory, you will find that not only has your conscious mind been at work, but your subconscious as well. If you have any prejudices (even those you hide from yourself), they will have bubbled up if the occasion arose. Surely you have heard people say, "He's a conceited son of a bitch" after a single meeting with someone to whom they may not have spoken two words. Consciously, they saw a man who stood, walked, or moved his hands in a given way, but subconsciously they registered a conceited son of a bitch out of their past who did one or all of those same things.

Because of this ability of the subconscious to put movement patterns and character traits together, Madison Avenue is able to keep us dancing to its tunes. Madison Avenue has taken the trouble to do exactly that. The head-up, straight-shouldered stance is rarely if ever presented by either a sick or unhappy person. Sickness, fear, anxiety, and misery, as well as a lack of self-confidence, present quite a different picture. The back is rounded, head droops, face sags, hands grip or wring each other or hide in pockets, arms clutch protectively across the chest, the shoulders hunch, and the abdomen protrudes.

Madison Avenue's sexually attractive male need not be six feet tall, but he must move with a catlike grace, his shoulders swinging free of tension, his back straight, and his abdomen flat. His springing walk says the world belongs to him, but his disarming smile says that since you are his friend you have an "in" in high places. The sexually attractive female need not measure up to what might be called either American Beauty standards or those set for California fruit. She does, however, step lightly with head high. Her breasts are not hidden behind clutching crossed arms that round the back and force loose abdominals forward. She has a tight little seat and well-made, well-muscled legs. When she runs it is with a fluid, efficient motion. Should she lean against anything, including the attractive male, it is with the most artfully balanced control, assuring you that the slightest disturbance, even just a whim of her own, would send her racing lightly across sand or meadow, leaving only laughter in her wake. Do you see those two pictures? Consciously you would find them pleasant to look at; subconsciously you would feel that both were in complete control. Both of those feelings sell products for Madison Avenue. Now, how does this apply to you?

Movement, anybody's, is like the weather map pictured each day on TV or in the paper. It tells all about what is going on everywhere right then *at that given moment*. It is also like a long-term report from a computer that has tracked the weather every single day for twenty years. The current map works this way to reveal your current mood.

Say you have just had words with your supervisor, your spouse, or the president of the company. You know you can't escape from the situation and have no recourse other than to stay and take it. What's more, you *know* you were right. What emotions will you feel? Self-righteousness, irritation, anger, and frustration. Later on we'll discuss the price you will have to pay for harboring such emotions, but right now let's look at your movement patterns. Anger clenches teeth and fists, gut and gluteals. Self-righteousness strains the chest forward and the shoulders back, frustration combines all of those things and adds something else that is worse than all the others combined. When you are completely frustrated, you give up fighting the outside influence and, like an animal with a leg caught in a trap, commence to gnaw on your own tissues. You may say all the agreeable words such as "Yes, yes indeed, I see your point . . ." but your body keeps flashing "I'd like to lam you one." When you turn and walk away, every inch of your unyielding back repeats that pronouncement. You look angry, you stand angry, and you walk angry. What's more, you will probably carry the whole mess around in stiff-muscled silence for the rest of the day.

Now let's take a different situation. You are caught in what seems to be a hopeless, overwhelming situation. It might be the loss of a loved one, it might be a devastated career, it might be grave financial reverses, even ruin. It might be any one of the thousand catastrophes that plague thousands of people any day in any city. Your sorrow will cause your shoulders to sag and your head to bow down. Your hands may clutch, clamp, or wring each other. You may hide them in your pockets or let them lie limp in your lap. If the doorbell rings, your quiet footfall and halting rhythm will advertise your condition even before your visitor catches sight of your weary body and strained face. Madison Avenue would have no use for either of those movement patterns. Neither anger nor sorrow sells anything.

Now let's look at what the long-term effect of emotions with their selective postural and movement patterns can show. Draw ten one-inch squares on a sheet of paper and label them, like this:

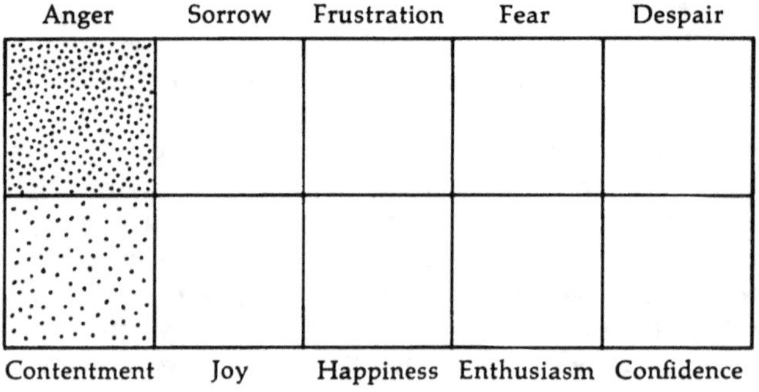

Anger	Sorrow	Frustration	Fear	Despair
Contentment	Joy	Happiness	Enthusiasm	Confidence

Now, imagine that over a twenty-year period the emotion that was dominant each day received from your computer *one dot of ink*—that's 7,300 dots. Now take your own pen and put 100 dots in just one of those boxes; 100 dots would represent 100 days, or 1.3% of your emotional states over twenty years. Now, carefully, without running one dot into another, place 300 dots (or 4%) of your possible emotional states in another box. If 4% of your emotional states were put into the Anger box, which your body would portray with hunched shoulders, tight facial muscles, clenched fists, and a stiff back, and 1% fell into the Contentment box with its relaxed muscles and sweet half-smile, what would your general posture and habitual expression be after twenty years?

Of course, nothing is quite that simple, but it certainly can show a trend, and as you will discover in the chapter on stress, it may tell you where your headaches are coming from. And for others it may reveal a source of something that is too often dismissed as frigidity and impotence.

The purpose of self-examination, whether the tests we make are to determine physical condition, mental outlook, emotional state, or even the quality of our lives, is to know exactly where we stand. The person who gets on a scale each morning knows the exact date when weight starts to rise. With such instant information, it is possible to do something easy and immediate to control the problem. The person whose weight remains constant year after year, but whose tape measure shows that it has slid down from chest to belly, is in possession of similar helpful information and will be able to get things under control before they have a chance to injure his or her self-image. The person who is brought up short by the realization that 320 out of 365 days in a single year have been filled with stress, misery, and despair may be wise enough to change the situation before one year has become five and the physical reactions to such unhappiness have become virtually irreversible.

This is a book about sexuality and everything that affects it: the way you spend your days, your physical condition, the people around you, the food you eat, and the atmosphere at the tables where you eat it. It is affected and even influenced by how often you play, what you play at, and where. It is not your age or how many orgasms you have (or even if you have any) that determines your level of sexuality. That potential was yours when you were born, and it is there now to be augmented, implemented, and, in some cases, recovered.

On the following pages you will meet yourself not as you may think you are, but as you really are. You may be in for some surprises that should be considered neither good nor bad, merely very interesting and significant. But if you wish to improve both your sex life and your life in general, the first step is to improve the house you live in, your body.

3

How Fit Is Fit?

Madison Avenue chooses its models not merely for their looks, but even more for the way they sit, stand, and move. These valuable assets are *controlled* by the strength and flexibility of key posture muscles, the abdominals, psoas (hip flexors), the upper and lower back muscles, and the hamstrings. Far more important to your level of sexuality than hair color, skin texture, or clothing size is the state of these muscles. They are the frame upon which you hang everything else. Every really healthy person can pass the following tests—all six of them. Height, weight, age, or length of legs has nothing to do with it. If your doctor told you that you had a perfectly clean bill of health except for that disturbing sound coming from your heart, you would not go your way rejoicing. Failure to pass means many things concerning your general well-being; where sex is concerned, it means that physically you could not carry out all the lovely things you have in mind. In other words, you might be where the action is—but there wouldn't be much of it.

The happy thing about these key muscles is that they respond to attention the way two lovers respond to each other—immediately, gratefully, willingly, and completely. There is an important difference. Sometimes love wanes and its duties become burdensome. With your muscles, this can never happen. There can be no waning of their need for care (nor of your need to care for them), and the more attention you lavish on them, the greater will be both response and reward. This is not one of those senseless exams concerning useless trivia you used to take in school. This is an important test about an important subject—you.

Minimum-Muscular-Fitness Test For Key Posture Muscles

Understand what each test is all about. We know too little about our bodies, and ignorance in such a vital area is dangerous to your well-being.

Test 1. Abdominals Plus Psoas (A+)

At the very bottom of the abdominal-strength ladder is a test we label A+ for *abdominals plus psoas or hip flexors*. Most people know where their abdominal muscles are but the psoas is for many a mystery muscle. It starts in the mid-back and runs down *inside* the pelvis, ending in the top of the thighs. The word is pronounced "so-az" and is defined as "a muscle of the loin, arising internally from the sides of the spinal column and fitting into the upper end of the thighbone." When both the abdominals and psoas are strong, half of all posture problems disappear; but sometimes, when the abdominals are weak, the psoas is forced to do more than its share of work. That puts considerable strain on the back, and a person with a "bad back" is usually a sexually handicapped person. Even when pain is absent, the possibility of the back "going out" during intercourse is not only a risk in itself but it becomes a presence in the subconscious and acts like a brake on free movement. One need not have weak abdominals to cause trouble by overworking a psoas. The men in the army who did hundreds of straight-leg sit-ups during basic training owe most of their aching backs to that exercise rather than to the heavy packs they carried. Many had been conditioned for trouble long before being inducted into the army by doing straight-leg sit-ups in high-school gym classes or as warm-ups before basketball or football practice.

To find out about the state of your abdominals and psoas, lie down on the floor with hands clasped behind your head, legs straight, and feet held down. Roll up to full sitting position only *once* and then roll back down. If you were able to do that, you have at least the beginnings of a good set of abdominals, which will not only serve you well sexually but in every other way, including appearance. Put a check after A+ in box A on page 35. If you couldn't sit up, or if you found it difficult, then you will find it impossible to get the most from your sex life, and you are certainly in danger of incurring a "bad back." If you flunked, enter a zero in your score box and think "Thank goodness!" One of the hardest things to endure is not knowing what to do about a problem, but you will soon know exactly what to do about this one. If you found the sit-up difficult, consider it as just about failed. It would be a failure if you had to spend much time sitting or if you were ever ill enough to need bed rest.

Test 2. Abdominals Minus Psoas (A−)

Test 2 is labeled A−, which stands for abdominals working without help from the psoas. You start as in test 1, supine with hands clasped behind your head, but this time you bend your knees. The person holding your feet down should exert plenty of pressure. With your knees bent you cannot put any strain on your back, you make it impossible for the psoas to get in the act, and since the abdominals must therefore do the whole job, there is no way for them to get out of working. This is not only the truer test for abdominals, it is also the only way to do safe sit-ups with hands clasped behind the head. If you can sit up once, put a check next to A− in Box A. If you couldn't sit up, give yourself a zero. That would put you in the same leaky boat with about 25% of our American schoolchildren, which is certainly a sad commentary on our schools. But imagine this: at least 43% of our little boys *enter* school at age six unable to sit up *once*, while only 2% of the little boys of Europe have that problem.

If you failed either or both of those abdominal tests, use the following exercises to repair yourself. But don't start your exercises until after you have taken your measurements (page 52), since one of the first rewards for labors performed will be a flatter abdomen.

1. Bent-knee Sit-ups

Start at the top of the sit-up position with hands clasped behind your head, knees bent, and feet weighted down, just as you did in the test. Roll *slowly* downward, trying to make each button of your spine touch separately. Sit up any way you can, and repeat. Do five roll-downs morning and night for two weeks and then retest.

If you are too weak to roll down slowly and under control, move your hands to the front and cross them over your chest while you roll down. Do the roll-downs in this fashion for one week and then try again with hands in back of your head. After two weeks, test again.

If you could sit up all right but held yourself stiff, as though there could be no bend in your back, then you were substituting or using muscles improperly. That is not the way the back should act, so put a check next to *substitution* in Box B. Do five roll-downs night and morning with head down, back rounded, and arms stretched straight forward. Try to *feel* each segment of spine as it touches the floor. In two weeks shift your hands to the cross-chest position and, as your ability to stay curved improves, shift the hands to behind your head.

If you managed to sit up in the abdominal tests but found that you twisted your torso so that one or the other elbow led either coming up or going down, you have uneven muscle development. Put a check next to *lead,* plus L for left or R for right. Then do your *roll-downs* every morning and night with the other elbow leading. In two weeks start sitting *up* with the same elbow leading.

After two weeks of these abdominal exercises, three things will have happened: your muscles will be stronger, your abdominals flatter, and your waist slimmer (if you didn't eat for two in the meantime).

Test 3. Psoas (P)

Test 3 is labeled P for psoas. That muscle was developed when you were a child if you were given the opportunity to walk a lot, run, skip, climb, and jump. However, the chances to do those things have declined steadily since 1930, when "calisthenics" became a naughty word and physical education gave itself over to a games program. 23% of our fourteen-year-old girls flunk this one, but *no* European girl of that age fails. If you fail, you can consider yourself sexually handicapped, but only for the three weeks of exercise it will take you to pass. You will need this muscle very badly when we come to pelvic tilts, which are considered basic for sexercise. Just remember where that muscle is—*inside the pelvis.*

Lie supine with legs straight. Lift both legs about ten inches above the floor and hold them there for ten seconds. You can count seconds by adding a three-syllable word to each number, as, one-chim-pan-zee, two-chim-pan-zees, etc. If you pass, put a check next to P in Box A. If you were not able to hold for the full count, enter the second that marked your touch-down.

You can pass the test but be in trouble all the same if your back arches unduly. If the psoas isn't strong enough, you will instinctively arch your back to shorten the muscle and make the lift easier. It is also possible that you have a sway back. If you find you do have more than a slight arch, but a check next to *arch* in Box B and, if you fail to hold for the full ten seconds, do the following exercise five times night and morning.

2. Spine Down-stretch

Lie supine and bend your knees to bring your thighs close to your abdomen. Slide your fingers under your back and make sure that it is pressed tight to the floor. *That's where it has to stay.* Extend both legs straight up, making sure there is no bend in the knees. Return to the bent-knee starting position. On the next extension, lower your legs a little closer to the floor. Check to see that your spine is still flat and then return to the starting position. Extend time and again, always a little lower, until you find you can no longer keep the spine down in contact with the floor. At that point return to the last extension when you could and do five. Repeat this exercise night and morning. Retest in two weeks. The final object is to be able to extend both legs about two inches above the floor while keeping the spine down. After that, if you wish to improve further, hang weight bags on each ankle (page 134).

It is important to understand that you cannot afford at any age to neglect any weakness or evidence of inflexibility. In the chapter "Pain—Preserver of Sexuality," you will see how a muscle deficiency can become chronic and lead to both premature and very uncomfortable symptoms of aging. Pain can interfere with your lovemaking as well as with your aura of healthy sexuality. If your car had tires that were wearing unevenly, you would check out your wheel balance. That's because you know that imbalance can cause irreparable damage. Be as kind, careful, and considerate with yourself.

Test 4. Upper Back (UB)

Test 4 is labeled UB for upper back. With the help of someone else's hands and eyes, this test can tell you a great deal about yourself.

Lie prone with your hands clasped behind your head. If your back is very inflexible or if your bust is large, place a pillow or rolled towel under your hips. The tester holds the person being tested with a hand across both calves. This leaves the other hand free for exploration. Lift your upper body so that it clears the floor, and hold for ten seconds. If you can hold the full count of ten, enter a check next to

UB in Box A. If you cannot hold for ten, enter the number of the second when you touched down. It is a rare person who fails this one. After all, at least *minimum* back strength is developed when we lean over to pick things up. However, passing or failing isn't all there is to this test. While you are holding the lift, the tester checks the two muscles running down either side of the spine to discover if one side is more developed than the other. By cupping the hand over the muscle on one side at the waist and then crossing over to cup the muscle on the other side, the tester can feel if one bulge is larger than the other. This cupping is repeated about every two inches all the way up the back. If one side is larger, it is an indication of an uneven development in the torso muscles and therefore of an uneven pull. It may also be an indication of spinal curvature, or *scoliosis*. Curvature usually begins during the growth spurt at about age eleven and then sets at its final curvature about age seventeen. It is well to know if you have scoliosis (many people do), because by its very presence it indicates an imbalance somewhere, and any imbalance left unattended can lead to fatigue and pain. Fatigue and pain are not aids to making love and may deter you from even wanting to. You will discover in test 6 whether or not you actually do have such a problem. In the meantime, if one side is larger than the other, indicate this next to *uneven* in Box B.

During the test, have the tester notice whether you stretch your elbows out wide, causing the upper back to flatten. This denotes good upper-back strength as well as plenty of stretch in the *pectorals*, or chest muscles. (Both men and women have them.) Gymnasts, dancers, and swimmers usually have fine flat upper backs. If the elbows droop downward, look for a round back or round shoulders when you get around to checking posture. To improve upper back strength, use exercise 3.

3. Back-lifts over a Box

Lie prone over a box padded with a pillow. The edge of

the bed will do almost as well. Rest arms on the floor and then, with feet held down, raise the upper body until it's at least level with the top of the box, farther if you can. Lower to the floor for a two-second rest and then repeat. Start with three lifts and gradually work up until you can do ten with ease. To further improve, add weight bags (page 134) to the back of your neck.

Test 5. Low back (LB)

Test 5 is labeled LB. Lie prone with head resting on folded arms. The tester places both hands in the middle of the upper back and presses down firmly as you lift your legs clear and hold them up for ten seconds. If you pass, put a check next to LB in Box A. If not, note the second of touch-down. Use exercise 4 to improve.

4. Leg-lifts over a Box

Lie prone over a padded box or bed edge. If you use a box, rest elbows on the floor. If you use the edge of the bed, rest arms on the bed. In either case, rest bent knees on the floor. With plenty of pressure applied to the upper back by your tester, raise straight legs until they are at least level with the rest of the body. Lower to the floor and repeat. Start with three and work up to ten. To further improve your performance, hang weight bags from the ankles.

While exercise 4 is excellent for the low back, it is also a good exercise to improve the size, shape, and strength of the *gluteals* (seat muscles). It is not hard to understand the value of these muscles in lovemaking. If the seat is flabby, even when it is not fat, it signals weakness and ineptitude. It also advertises lack of practice.

Test 6. Flexibility (Flex)

Text 6 is labeled flex for back and hamstring flexibility. This is the only test for flexibility in the entire *minimum* test battery. It is, however, as important and revealing as all the others put together. The usual cause of inflexibility in the back and hamstrings (the muscles running down the backs of the legs) is a lack of sufficient physical outlet to balance emotional stress and accumulated tension. Such inflexibility can also be caused by poor coaching in sports, but since 53% of our seven-year-old boys (who have not yet even seen a coach) flunk the test, one has to believe that it is our way of life that is to blame. Only 3% of Europe's seven-year-olds fail in this area.

Do not warm up for this test. Place your feet together and keep your knees straight. Bend forward *slowly* from the hips, reaching downward with straight arms. See how close you can bring your fingertips to the floor. Hold at your farthest reach for three seconds. If you can touch, you pass. Put a T for *touch* in Box A next to *flex*. Barely touching isn't great, but it counts as a pass. A few weeks under pressure—without sufficient physical outlet—and you would fail. If you can't even touch, enter in minus inches the distance between fingers and floor. To improve, do exercise 5.

5. Flexibility Bounces

There are two positions for your bounces. Start with legs widespread and hands clasped behind your back. *Keeping your head up,* bounce your upper body downward eight times. Then drop arms, head, and upper body down, letting them hang loose. Bounce downward again eight times. *Don't push.* Just let gravity do the work, while you concentrate on *feeling* where the tight spots are, and try to let go. Stress and tension are always with us, so the cure for inflexibility must be invoked as often as possible throughout the day. Do three sets of the bounces as often as you can. Do them in or after your shower, and before you leave for work or start your chores at home. Do them in the lavatory midmorning, before or after lunch, midafternoon, before dinner, and before bed. Do them whenever the sports news flashes on TV. *And when things are rough, do more of them.* Inflexibility in those areas is a prime cause of backache, and usually at the most inconvenient time. The silliest-looking man in the world is the fellow who hobbles into the doctor's office on Monday morning with his back in an agonizing spasm. Where did he get it? "In bed, Doc!"

Before we leave this area, add one more thing to your test. The quickest way to spot scoliosis, or curvature of the spine, is with the same action used in test 6. As you lean *slowly* downward, the tester stands behind you and, stooping so as to keep his eyes level with your bending back, watches as the descent is made. If the two sides of the back stay level all the way down, there is no scoliosis. If, however, one side seems to rise higher than the other at *any time during the descent,* then you do have scoliosis. To discover which side of your back is limited in movement, stand with feet apart and arms extended straight out to the sides at shoulder level. Pretend you are in a closet, and keeping arms level and legs stiff, try to touch the imaginary walls, first on one side and then on the other. You will be able to reach farther on one side, so it is the other side that will need "closet-wall reaches" several times each day.

If you are an adult and find that you have scoliosis, it would be helpful if you would do as many bilateral exercises as you can. These would be such things as rowing, swimming, gymnastics, or just plain sexercises. While the curvature is "set"—and not likely to go further—there is still a certain amount of imbalance and your muscles were not designed for the strain this imposes. The exercises will prevent further tightening, shortening, and limitation of movement due to pain.

If the test is done on a youngster between the ages of eleven and seventeen, it would be worthwhile to consult a doctor for a more vigorous and specific program of exercise.

Optimum Fitness

There is probably a level of fitness that might be called optimum, but no one has ever attained it. We use only about one-fifth of our mental abilities in a world that is constantly demanding that we exercise our brains. The same world calls for an absolute minimum of physical action from most of us, and because this is so, we develop very little of our physical potential indeed. *If* we were to set up a program that increased the demands on our bodies a little more each year, we would continue to improve physically (and therefore sexually) as we grew older and older. But what do we do? We are forced into sedentary lives as children by a way of life that prevents us from being active and close to nature. We are kept sedentary as teenagers and young adults, and a little later we cheerfully embrace inactivity as we lose the spark of vitality we brought with us into the world. When we view our flabby, sometimes spindly, often obese bodies, we moan pitifully about aging. Had we the wit to view Michelangelo's mightily muscled graybeards as models taken from life, we might wonder if things were once different, and perhaps better.

The tragedy of our enforced deterioration is that it need never take place. If you will set up your *sexercise* program right now, there isn't a reason in the world why you should ever join the ranks of the "elderlies" who "don't anymore."

I was once deeply in love with a man who said to me, "If we part, will you hate me?" Shocked to my soul, I asked, "Have you fallen out of love with me?" "Oh, no," he answered. "Don't think such a thing for a minute. It is only when such a possibility is impossible that one can discuss it without discomfort." It is only while you are young, strong, healthy, and in love with love that you can view with detachment the possibility that one day you will not be young. It is now, while everything is going your way, that you must take steps to ensure that it will continue this way. If you are going to make a few more demands on your body each year from this day forward, you will need to know just how good you are right now in order to ensure constant improvement. You already know if you are below minimum levels of fitness, and if you are, you also know that in a few weeks you can be ready to take on some of the more difficult tests and exercises. You may already be in shape, but lacking in one or another area. If you do not have the necessary flexibility but do have the required strength, go forward into the following optimum tests wherever you can and bring the lagging areas along. Just don't work your good muscles and neglect the ones that need extra help.

No two people in any one family will have the same score when it comes to optimums, and that should make no difference at all. It is not necessary to do better than the next fellow even if he is your twin. Each person's individual score sets the level of competition. You need not be better or best when it comes to others, but you *must* be better next year than you are today, and if you will work at it, there isn't a way in the world you can fail.

Optimum Tests

Test 7. Abdominals (ABD)

Test 7 is labeled ABD for abdominals. If you passed tests 1 and 2, you are ready for the next step. Often, determining the optimum strength of the abdominals is done by doing as many sit-ups as possible. This is invariably followed by several days of muscle soreness in the abdominal area and, for some people, skin abrasion at the base of the spine. It is not an experience one elects to repeat. There is, however, a quicker, easier, simpler, and painless way to obtain the desired information.

Take the same bent-knee position used in test 2. This time, however, you will be doing sit-ups against resistance. The most accurate way to check both your optimum level of abdominal strength and your rate of improvement is to use weight bags (page 134). A versatile set would contain two one-pounders, two two-pounders, and two five-pounders. If the man of the house is in good shape, you should add a second set of five-pounders to be used in the weight-training section (pages 46–60). To test, take the bent-knee position with one one-pound weight held in both hands behind your neck. With feet held down, roll up to the sitting position and then roll down again. On the second sit-up, hold a two-pound bag behind your neck. On the third hold a two-pounder plus a one-pounder, on the fourth two two-pounders. Keep on increasing a pound with each sit-up until you can no longer get your back off the floor to do even one more. Enter the poundage carried in the last successful sit-up under ABD in Box C. Then, for the next *month*, do ten sit-ups night and morning with one-half your maximum lift. Then retest. You will be flatter, stronger, and in greater control of the pelvis.

Not everyone can get together a set of weight bags, but everyone can find either a heavy book or a rock. The weight, whatever it is, should be heavy enough to make more than ten sit-ups almost impossible, but five at least bearable. To improve, do half the maximum number of lifts twice a day, oftener if possible. Keep track of the number of lifts you do and also the number of times you lift. For example, four lifts or sit-ups done four times a day should be written up as 4 × 4. In time, when you can test out with the same weight and sit up sixteen times, your homework would be written up as 8 × 4. When you can sit up twenty times with that weight, you need a heavier weight! To hurry improvement, do exercise 6.

6. Sit-ups over a Box

Sit on a padded box with feet held down. Extend both hands in front and roll *slowly* down until your head and shoulders are *resting* on the floor. Extend both arms overhead and then swing them forward, allowing the momentum to carry you up into the sit-up position. When you feel strong enough, roll down with arms crossed over your chest, and then, using the overhead swing, sit up. In time, try to roll down with hands behind your head and sit up with arms crossed over your chest. Still later, roll down and up again with hands behind your head. Start with a small number and work up. For a heavy workout, carry a weight in your hands.

Test 8. Push-ups (PU)

Test 8 is labeled PU for push-ups. If you know you can do a few push-ups, take the prone position, lying *feet together* with hands placed on the floor just outside of your shoulders. Keeping your body rigid, push up to full arm stretch and lower slowly, taking five full seconds for the descent. Be sure to maintain the rigidity of your body. After reaching the floor, lift both hands and bring them around to touch over your back. Repeat the exercise a second time and a third, until you can do no more. Enter the number of correct push-ups (body rigid and raised to full arm stretch with five-second lowering) under PU in Box C. If you find the push-ups with feet together too demanding, try them with legs spread wide. Observe the same conditions: body rigid, full arm stretch, five-second lowering and then touching hands over your back before going on. Enter your score. In both cases, do one-half the optimum number every day. The reason you lower slowly and then touch hands over your back is that you want to force your muscles to work all along their full length. The initial lift from the floor is very demanding, just as getting anything moving from a standstill is far more difficult than just keeping it moving once it is in motion. The first inch of lift off the floor calls for more effort than all the rest of the lift to full arm stretch.

What about the person who can't do even one? No, it's not because of your sex or your build; it's because you lack strength in your arms and chest and shoulders. It wouldn't take a "how-to" book to see how that might limit your pleasure when making love. Start at the top of the push-up position with legs well spread. Keeping your body rigid, lower yourself *slowly* until you rest at full length on the floor. Touch your hands together over your back (to establish a pattern) and then get back up any way you can and as far as you can and repeat the descent. Do five lowerings night and morning for a month and then retest. You'll be pleasantly surprised.

Test 9. Chin-ups (CU)

Test 9 is labeled CU for chin-ups. Get a chinning bar at a sports store and install it in the frame of the bathroom door. Do not trust the kind that relies entirely on suction cups to keep it in place. They have been known to let go, with painful results, especially when used by tall men who must bend their knees to clear the floor when at full hang. Brace the bar with small angle irons.

The test is made up of two parts, the first for the *biceps,* the muscles in the front of your upper arms. Hang at full length from the bar with palms facing toward your body. Pull yourself up until your chin is even with the bar. Lower slowly, taking five full seconds for the descent. Then step away from the bar and reverse the direction of your hands so that the palms face away from your body. This will test the *triceps* in the backs of your upper arms. Do a second chin-up in this position. Alternate hands, doing as many chin-ups as you can. Enter your final result under CU in Box C and do one-half your maximum number of lifts each day, night and morning. One more thing. Never go through that door again without doing a palms-*in* chin-up as you go in and a palms-*out* chin-up as you go out. This is a painless way to improve the strength of arms, chest muscles, and shoulders, and to improve a bust line.

And what if you can't do a single chin-up? You do *let-downs.* Using a box, a chair, or a jump-up-pull-up, start at the top of the chin-up with palms facing in. Let yourself slowly down, trying to control the descent for *ten* full seconds (you won't be able to at first, it will be more like three). Then reverse your hands and repeat the slow let-down. When you can let down slowly enough to require ten seconds, you will have the strength to do at least one chin-*up.* You too should use the chin-up password to get into and out of the bathroom all day long.

Test 10. Broad Jump (BJ)

Test 10 is labeled BJ for broad jump, and it tests the explosive power of your legs. If you are interested in sexuality, you should be interested in both the strength and appearance of your legs. Even a cursory look at the "how-to" manuals will tell you that the day (or night) of passivity and detachment in lovemaking is past. While you have no intention of jumping from the doorway into the center of your bed, you should have legs that could, if you chose to, do exactly that. Just knowing you have that sort of power is of psychological value.

Pin a tape measure to the living-room rug (if it's wall-to-wall and non-skid). Or, using rubber cement, you can glue it to the floor in the hall or kitchen. Stand next to it at one end (if you can jump farther than six feet, which is the length of the average household tape measure, step back two feet and add twenty-four inches to your final score) and get set to jump. Getting set means standing with feet apart, knees bent, arms back, and body leaning forward. When you jump, fling your arms forward to assist. Try three jumps and enter your best score under BJ in Box C. Measure from the starting line to the heel of the nearest foot.

If you have never done such a thing, or if several years have passed since you did, be content with small beginnings. Don't be discouraged if you lack spring. It isn't what you do today that counts, but what you will be doing a month from today. Be aware that your feet, legs, gluteals, psoas, and abdominals aren't *yet* performing very well either in concert or as soloists. If you can, leave the tape right there and make a point of jumping every chance you get, even if you don't try for all-out performance. *Any* jump is better than no jump, and *any* jump done ten times a day is bound to get results.

Test 11. Flexibility Plus (FP)

Test 11 is labeled FP for flexibility plus. If you passed

test 6 for *minimum* flexibility, as about 50% of you should have, you are now ready to find out how much better than barely flexible you are. Stand on a box or on a chair and, with feet together and knees straight but *without any warm-up*, lean down and see how far your fingers will reach beyond the stand platform. Be sure to have your results checked with a ruler and enter your results as plus inches under FP in Box D. To improve, stand on that same platform with either weight bags or a couple of heavy books in your hands. Do the flexibility bounces (exercise 5), allowing gravity plus the added weight in your hands to stretch your back and hamstring muscles. Do about sixteen bounces twice a day *after you have warmed up with other exercises.*

Test 12. Crotch Flexibility (CF)

Test 12 is labeled CF for crotch flexibility. Tight muscles in the crotch are a definite handicap when it comes to lovemaking and for a great many other activities as well. It is quite true that you may have been doing quite well (as far as you know) without this valuable asset, but then you may feel that way because you don't know what you are missing. That's not really a good reason for ignoring the possibilities. To find out about your advantage or limitation, draw your feet up close to your body and place them sole to sole. Grasp your ankles with your hands and press your elbows down on both knees. Keep the pressure even and measure the distance from the floor to the center of one kneecap. Enter the measurement as minus inches under CF in Box D. A minus three inches would be almost perfect, a minus twelve would be awful. What it is today is merely your take-off point, but what it is in a month will be important. To improve, sit in the test position and press down hard. Hold for ten seconds and release. While you are holding, sit with closed eyes, trying to *feel* where the muscles are tight, and relax them. Do this at least twice a day, and oftener if you can manage. The crotch, like the back and hamstrings, is a tension target; since tension is with us always, we should remember to protect the areas most affected by it.

Test 13. Low-back Flexibility (LBF)

Test 13 is labeled LBF for low-back flexibility. The lower back, like the crotch, plays an important part in lovemaking and is also a tension target. Draw your feet close to your body and place them sole to sole. Grasping the ankles, try to bring your head down to rest on your feet. If you can touch, you can be sure of excellent low-back flexibility. If you can't (and age has nothing to do with it; it is caused by tight back muscles), it is something you should work for very hard. Tight back muscles force you to move awkwardly, lift heavy objects incorrectly, and tire easily. They can also lead straight to a very painful back condition which will limit you in anything you want to do, from sitting at your typewriter to what you are using this book for. Give yourself T for touch, or indicate any minus inches by which you fail to touch under LBF in Box D. To improve, pull your head down in sixteen easy bounces, trying to *feel* the tight places, and let go. Do this several times and at least twice a day.

When either crotch flexibility or low-back flexibility improves, it should be heralded with champagne or a reasonable facsimile. Any strain in these areas can cause discomfort. No one is at his best when under strain, and there is always the danger that a warning flicker of pain will intrude. This can present as much inhibition as the possibility of intrusion by another person.

Test 14. Soleus Stretch (SS)

Test 14 is labeled SS for soleus stretch (heel-cord stretch), and you may feel like asking, "What have my heel cords got to do with my love life?" Nothing at the moment, if you are under thirty. But a youthful gait, like a youthful waistline, is important both to appearance and to your self-image. Strength and flexibility of feet and ankles will protect that self-image against shortened steps and an unconscious unwillingness to stoop down and pick things up. That particular self-limitation will sooner or later lead to weakened quadriceps (thigh muscles), with accompanying flabbiness where none can be afforded.

Stand facing a wall without a baseboard. If there is no such wall, use a broomstick or pole to provide the vertical limitation. With feet together, pelvis tucked under, and toes pointing straight forward about two inches from the wall or pole, bend both knees to touch it if you can. If you fail to touch with both knees (if one has been injured, make a note of it and test them separately), move a little closer and try again. If your knees touch with ease *while heels are held tight to the floor,* move your feet farther away. Five inches could be considered good and one inch very poor. To improve, use exercise daily. Use that exercise often, even if you feel quite pleased with your test results. Whenever we are under pressure, we tense muscles, and when we forget to stretch them, they have a tendency to stay tight—which ultimately shortens them. *All* your muscles need stretching, and foot muscles need this as much as any.

A	B	C	D
A+	arch lead substitution uneven	ABD	FP
A−	arch lead substitution uneven	PU	CF
P	arch lead substitution uneven	CU	LBF
UB	arch lead substitution uneven	BJ	SS
LB	arch lead substitution uneven		
flex	arch lead substitution uneven		

4

A Lovely Way to Go ... But Not for You

Whenever love is being made, four partners are involved—two people and two hearts. It is not for nothing that every valentine wears a heart. It is not from lack of imagination or because of anatomical ignorance that poets give their hearts to loved ones. Without the cooperation of hearts, love would be denied one of its most meaningful facets. One of the very first signs that love has entered in is the sudden increased tempo of the beating heart. That increase may be so slight that even *you* are unaware of it, but not so your body. Every part of you, from your adrenals to the sweat glands in the palms of your hands, begins to agitate in varying degrees. During the act of love itself, the hearts enter into the joyous occasion with such enthusiasm that they beat harder than they would if asked to support jogging for two miles, riding more miles than that on a bike, racing to catch a bus, or even climbing five flights of stairs.

If your heart is in shape for three sets of tennis or a fast swim out to Half-Mile Rock, you probably never give a thought to its wild gyrations when lovemaking takes over. Make no mistake about that. You may initiate the first stages, but after a certain point, you lose that control and there is little you can do except go forward with ever-mounting waves of excitement. Even if you aren't in very good shape, it is unlikely that you will question your partner-heart as to its condition and ability to stand the strain. Almost nobody, once the delightful confusion begins, thinks of anything other than the delightful confusion—unless of course you or a loved one has had and survived a heart attack.

They do say that, since we all have to die sometime anyway, dying of a quick heart attack while making love is a lovely way to go. Nonsense! A heart attack is scary enough if it happens at your desk, on a plane, in the car, on the golf course, or even in your doctor's office. To have one while making love is the worst way to go, or almost go. It frightens *everyone* horribly, and the memory of that dreadful interruption haunts even the loveliest moments forever more. Since a heart attack is something to avoid at *any* time—and since, yes, it *can* be avoided—this could be the most important chapter you've read in this or any other year. To prevent such an occurrence and to be assured of long life and good loving, you need to know something about hearts and about the situation in which you live.

Not too long ago, in the early 1900's, heart attacks, which cause over half of our deaths yearly and in younger and younger men (women seem to be almost immune until menopause), were comparatively rare. That certainly suggests that heredity isn't involved in most instances. This ought to reassure those whose close relatives have keeled over in the prime of life. Since parents have been with us from the time of Adam and Eve, but coronary occlusion is a relatively recent addition to our problems, something either must have been added to our way of life or subtracted, something that makes it different for today's generation. The answer is both—addition and subtraction. In fact, we have added one thing, subtracted a second, augmented a third, and transformed a fourth . . . and there is something to be done about each one if you know the score.

1. *We have added pollution.* Pollution, whether it is in the form of the cigarette *you* smoke, the one the other person smokes, the stuff belched from factory stacks, coughed from the exhaust pipes of automobiles, seeped into our rivers and lakes or added to our food and drink, is *poison.* Pollution in any form is foreign to our bodies and puts a strain on our hearts.

2. *We have subtracted physical action,* both in our

work and in our play. It is no longer *necessary* to use our bodies in order to put food into our mouths and a roof over our heads. Babies start their lives (and their heart problems) in high chairs, playpens, strollers, car seats, and supermarket carts. Right from the beginning, they form sedentary patterns and lazy attitudes. Then, from the time they start school, it's all downhill, but in a bus. Real physical education, as it is known in other countries, such as Scandinavia, Russia, China, and even England, is virtually nonexistent for American children. Instead, our children are subjected to constant restraint, whether in conveyance or in classroom. This unnatural restraint of young growing animals goes on all day, five days a week. Saturday and Sunday are also lost for most of them. Ever-increasing traffic makes highways unsafe. Increased population has eaten up the fields, meadows, and woodlands to feed its need for housing and business. Lawless elements have forced more and more children to stay indoors so that their families know where they are, not just at ten o'clock at night, but every day after school and on weekends, from rising to retiring. To make such limitation of freedom bearable, children have free access to the mind-numbing programs presented on TV. Sitting with glazed eyes and slack jaws, they are finally molded into a slumped posture and attitude of acceptance to every weird and often violent idea presented. Instead of being the prime leaders in creative play, which breeds self-reliance, they rely on a button to entertain them, interest them, and excite them.

This new and unnatural way of life also fosters hordes of hyperactive, frantically jigging children who can neither control nor direct their energies. Instead of alternating hard work with rest, their hearts are called upon to bang away with the speed needed for an endless jogging session, day after exhausting day—unless they are quieted with drugs, which are another form of pollution.

3. *We have not only augmented the natural stresses of life, for which the healthy body is well prepared and equipped, we have multiplied them hundreds of times, for which we are neither equipped nor prepared.*

In the long-ago early 1900's, when heart attacks were rare, life wasn't so hectic, and there was a lower level of personal expectancy. In the first place, there weren't so many *things* money could buy, and men didn't have to push themselves so hard to provide for their family's *wants*, which are not to be confused with *needs*. There was no television in those days to whet the appetites of one half by showing them how the other half lived (even though up to their eyeballs in debt in order to maintain it). Anxiety didn't ride into most homes on the first of each month, when excesses encouraged by credit cards and charge accounts and buying on time took their toll. People had a greater sense of security. Most lived in large, multi-generation groups, and the feeling of safety that surrounded them was far more satisfying than the lonely togetherness of today's nuclear family.

Papa, who only occasionally turned out to be a tyrant or a ne'er-do-well, was far more often a hard-working, God-fearing man who demanded and got respect. Mama was somebody special, and she earned every bit of the love and respect she was accorded. The image of the American male as a bumbling, myopic half-man had not yet been flashed on the screen, nor had Mama lost her halo in the Ms. mists. Family discipline, school discipline, and church discipline were strong, and good examples were to be found in all three places. Children did not have to depend on their peers for direction. When decisions had to be made, one person may have had the last word but he didn't have to undergo the stress caused by total and lonely responsibility. It was spread across many willing and able shoulders.

There were fewer people in the world in those days and they weren't constantly jostling each other in corridors, stepping on each other's toes in elevators, or squashing against each other in buses, trains, and planes. And there was time. The stress of overloaded schedules and the tyranny of the clock were unknown to most people . . . and there was quiet. You could stop what you were doing whenever you felt like it and listen to the silence. True, there was many a shout of "Alley alley in free . . ." in the cool of the evening just before the children were called in for bed, but you didn't have to share the day with jackhammers, power saws, electric drills, welding torches, cars, buses, trucks, and planes, nor the night with someone else's radio, TV, and family fight. The Third and Sixth Avenue els rumbled, to be sure, but only on two streets in America.

The stress of keeping up with the man at the next desk or the woman in the next house or the kids in the next block was minimal. Average folk were content with their own accomplishments, and it wasn't a crime to be "average." The average man and woman of long ago could take pride in accomplishment. Dining was still an art form rather than an interruption in TV viewing. People worked at doing, making, and finishing things they could stand back from and admire. The assembly line, secretary pool, teaching from "units," and preparing a meal from three frozen blocks of "convenience" were as yet unknown.

Sometimes men and women had to decide whether or not to marry because they were faced with the stress of bringing what would turn out to be a seven-month baby into the world, but the stress of determining just who the father was or whether or not they could get back into the tenth grade after the baby was born came to very few. The stress of deciding between the risk of venereal disease and being thought "queer" is new to the world, and so is the stress attacking those who either will or won't go to the pot party, the pill party, or the sex party.

Kids have always had chips on their shoulders, but how often in history was the chip knocked off by another kid's zip gun along *with* the shoulder? The stress of living in cities where such things are commonplace is extreme indeed.

Keys have always been available, but this is a time when keys must be backed up with multiple locks, alarms, and various other protective devices. The stress connected with constant anxiety and unrelenting fear is damaging to nerves, digestion, and hearts.

4. *We have transformed food into dollars for manu-*

facturers and malnourishment for ourselves. Anytime a body is malnourished, that body suffers damage. Fatigue is a product of malnourishment, and it robs the body of the energy needed for productive work and play. Depression is a product of malnourishment, and depression steals all the joy from living. The inability to protect the body against the invasion of disease is a product of malnourishment, and that leaves the body open to misery, pain, and even death. When malnourishment is suffered by children, bodies and brains cannot develop properly. Growth is stunted, posture ruined, the ability to learn limited. When malnourishment is suffered by young adults, their level of work and, therefore, accomplishment is low. Their ability to produce healthy children is nonexistent and their sex drive, sensitivity, and endurance are of poor quality with resultant frustration. Their appearance and self-image are of a very low order, falling far below the requirements that TV, movies, and magazines assure them they must meet. When the sufferers try to brighten lackluster lives by resorting to drugs and the abuse of alcohol, they merely hasten their own deterioration. When malnourishment is suffered by older adults, the aging process is speeded, degenerative disease finds ground for its growth, and death comes early. When hearts are malnourished, they quit.

We used to think that only the poor were malnourished, and so they are. But today, even the wealthiest stand a good chance of suffering from poor nutrition. Unless you have been very aware of the changes in food sources, food distributors, food processing, and even in food structure, you are like a lamb wandering innocent and helpless among a bunch of slavering wolves. In Chapter 12 there are some plain facts you can use for your protection, and if you want a full life and a long one you had best start to be aware that you are (even in bed) what you eat.

Knowing that your heart is endangered by these four changes in our lives is probably the best insurance for you and yours that you can adopt a course that will keep you safe from heart attacks. You *know* that pollution is damaging. You *know* where its level is high, and you also know where it is low. What measures could you take to protect yourself? If you must stay where it is at its worst and there is no way out, then you will have to see that at least the other three threats cannot touch you. You, your body, and your heart will have enough trouble handling the one you cannot do anything about. Read the chapter on vacations carefully. Perhaps there are escape hatches you have never noticed. The thing you certainly can handle is physical activity. Chapter 13 may offer valuable suggestions on how you might best spend some leisure time, but if you did nothing more than follow the sexercise program you would be well protected. The chapter that deals with stress will help you assess the stresses in your life-style and provide you with some ways to handle mounting tension and keep it under control. There are some stresses from which you cannot escape, but there are many you need only recognize to disarm. There are others you cannot constantly endure . . . and live. Know the difference between them. The chapter on diet and nutrition will provide you with some valuable information on keeping the food processor's hand out of your pocket and his "convenient" nonfoods out of your arteries.

Knowing that inactivity, poor nutrition, the proliferation of polluting substances, and an ever-rising level of stress have broken millions of hearts is like knowing your house has termites. If you *do* something about the situation right now, you can control it and then enjoy your house fully. If you ignore it, one day the piano may fall through the riddled floor into the cellar, along with the pianist.

What do you really know about your tireless heart-partner, the one that by its condition will determine the quality of your life and could certainly determine the length of your life? To begin with, it is a muscle, and if it's healthy, you simply can't exhaust it. I have heard mothers warning their children not to do this or that because they would "strain" their hearts. These mothers are unaware that those running legs would sag limply to the ground, those lifting backs and arms would be completely incapable of bending, lifting, or holding long, long before the strongly beating hearts would give out. It is not the exercised heart that is in danger, nor even the overexercised heart that signals its condition with hammer blows that can even be seen in temple and neck pulses. No, it is the *unexercised* heart that is in peril. Like all other muscles, the heart will deteriorate when not called upon regularly to put forth extra effort over and above that called for in just getting through a day. This danger does not exist for the laborer, the athlete, the mountaineer, or the professional scuba diver. The hearts of such people get fine regular exercise, but most of us do not. A game of golf on Saturday afternoon, the occasional game of handball or volley ball during the week, five ski weekends a year, a fall hike up your state's highest mountain, cannot be called regular or even demanding exercise. This is especially true if you sit at a desk under considerable pressure five days a week for fifty weeks a year—and that's what most of us do. Taking care of a house and children doesn't provide it either. If you think it does, go to the park and look over the condition of most of the young housewives sitting there. One close look and you'll *know* they don't get exercise!

You need to know the shape of your heart right now, and you need to know how hard it must work to accomplish the tasks you are going to set before it. The better its condition, the less effort it needs to make, and that means fewer beats per minute. You also need to know how long it goes on working at top speed *after* the task is done before it slows down to a normal rate. The better the condition, the quicker the return. The average male heart beats 72 times a minute, the hearts of the average female and child a little faster. The athlete in top condition may have a heartbeat as slow as 40 beats a minute because his stronger heart is more efficient. However, your interest should not lie with *his* heart, but with your own, and it is *your* pulse that will figure in the following test.

Add the following score sheet to your record and take this test each month as you repeat the others. Don't guess about the condition of your heart. *Know.*

HEART CHECK

Date	At rest	Standing	Action	After 1 min.	After 5

Lie flat and rest completely for ten minutes and then take your pulse. The easiest way is to lay the tips of your fingers on your larynx or voice box. Then, if you are using your right hand, lift your fingers off the larynx and slide them about an inch to the right into the soft tissue of the neck, to rest on the pulsing artery. There is a pulse in your thumb which might confuse things. Don't use it. Use your fingers and count your heartbeat for a full minute. Enter your resting pulse under At Rest. Stand up and take it again, but this time for only fifteen seconds. Multiply the beat by four and enter it under Standing. Next, you want to know how it behaves when you put it under a little pressure. In the course of one minute you should be able to step up onto a box with first one foot and then the other, and then step down the same way, thirty times. If you are in *very* poor shape, or recovering from an accident or illness, be satisfied with fifteen times in half a minute. Take two full seconds for each up-down action, which consists of four separate steps. On the word "one," step up on the right foot. On the word "and," bring the left foot to the platform. On the word "two," step back down with the right foot, and on the word "and," bring the left down to the floor. When you have done thirty, take your pulse immediately for one full minute and enter the results under Action. The time required to take your pulse will have afforded you a one-minute rest period, so as soon as you have entered the Action pulse, take your pulse again, this time for fifteen seconds. Multiply the results by four and enter under After One Minute. Sit down and rest for five minutes and take it once more, using the fifteen-second–multiply-by-four system. Enter your results under After Five Minutes. Let me explain why you test this way.

Oxygen Debt

When your body is being very active, oxygen is burned at a much faster rate than can be replaced in the body right then and there. No matter how fast you breathe while the action is going on; you cannot replace all the oxygen you are using because your body can't absorb it fast enough. You go into what is called *oxygen debt.* Since you have already used up all the oxygen you had free in your body, you borrow from your own tissues with the tacit understanding that you will pay it back with a lot of fast panting when the action has been terminated.

It's like setting out on a trip and suddenly running out of money. You wire home to your brother, who lends you what you need until a time when you can find work, earn the money, and pay it back.

Naturally, if you are in good shape, you will be able to pay your debt quickly and efficiently. The debt itself won't be so great, because, since your circulation, lungs, and heart are good, you would have more free oxygen available at the start. As the months pass and you keep to your sexercise program, you will be improving your heart action, lung capacity, and your circulation. You will soon find that your heart returns to normal faster than it did at the start. In time, your starting pulse will be slower. There will be many other changes in your body, but this one has a very direct bearing on your lovemaking as well as all the rest of your life.

Your body is your vehicle, and it takes you where you want to go and permits you to do what you want to do. Your heart is the pump that fuels your vehicle. If it isn't equal to the demands you put upon it, you have what might be called a lemon of a vehicle. Making love can and should be very demanding physically. If you are too tired to look for love, that's a pity. However, if you are too tired to make love *when you are in love,* that's a disaster. It isn't the addition of years that makes people discontented with their sex lives; that is due more often than not to the loss of muscle tone from their hearts.

5

Off, Off, Damned Spot!

Most people judge their weight by the scale, but the only thing the scale reports accurately is the given weight of an individual at a given point in time, and that is but a small part of the whole story. A human being is not a homogeneous blob enclosed in a bag made of skin. We each possess a bony framework of different height, size, and density. Strapped over this frame, enabling it to remain erect, change position, and move from place to place, are numerous muscles. While we all have the same number of muscles, they vary greatly in size, weight, quality, and strength. Inside our supporting and protecting frames are organs. Here, too, we are alike only in numbers and kinds of organs. Their size, weight, and condition vary greatly. Then, in areas all over our bodies, we have deposits of fat—and in the unhappy realm of fat we do indeed differ, not only from one another but even from ourselves at different times.

The scale will tell us about the weight of the whole, but the tape measure will tell a great deal more. Fat weighs less than muscle, and in our society, a good proportion of the fat we accumulate is not only superfluous and unsightly, it is dangerous as well. While muscle is useful and attractive, it does weigh more—which could confuse you. Let's say that you wanted to shape up and you certainly needed to get rid of fifteen pounds. You started your overall exercise program with the best will in the world and you cut your usual number of calories by 500 a day. At the end of the month, when you got on your scale, it registered two pounds heavier. Unless you were in the know, you might panic. Then, there's the opposite side of the coin. You are too thin so you decide to try to improve things as Charles Atlas once did. You will start a graduated program of weight training, but because you know that weight training without stretch exercise can shorten muscles, and is inadequate without running or some similar taxing activity, you add those elements. By the end of the week you've lost a pound and a half, and if you are a woman you may find that your not overfilled bra is even baggier than usual. Panic again. In both cases, had you taken the trouble to measure yourself, you would have learned good news. In the first instance, though your muscles had improved in strength and tone, you were slimmer all over, fat having been melted away. Only good can come of that. The thin person would have to be a little patient; it is easier to lose fat (even the fat you want to keep) than to build up muscle. That will take time, but it is inevitable. If you are a woman, you need not fear that those muscles you are building will have a masculine quality. Only hormones can do that, as the delicate little dancers and gymnasts of the world have shown.

It is cheering to note that fat exits most readily from the abdominals (do exercise 1), which might be called the "pot," and from the waist (do exercise 8), which might be called the "tire." The message sent by the improving muscles is that not only are you getting to them, but to your circulation, skin tone, glands and organs, emotions, concentration, and endurance as well. Everything about you will receive at least some bonus for your efforts.

But while fat seems to disappear quite readily from some areas, it is extremely resistant in others. These stubborn areas all seem to double as target areas for emotional stress and tension. Quite unconsciously, whenever we are under pressure, we tighten certain parts of our bodies. Sometimes this repeated contraction of given muscles results in pain, such as backache, headache, stiff necks, and leg cramps. Sometimes there is no pain, but the target areas thicken and trap fat, leading to figure problems.

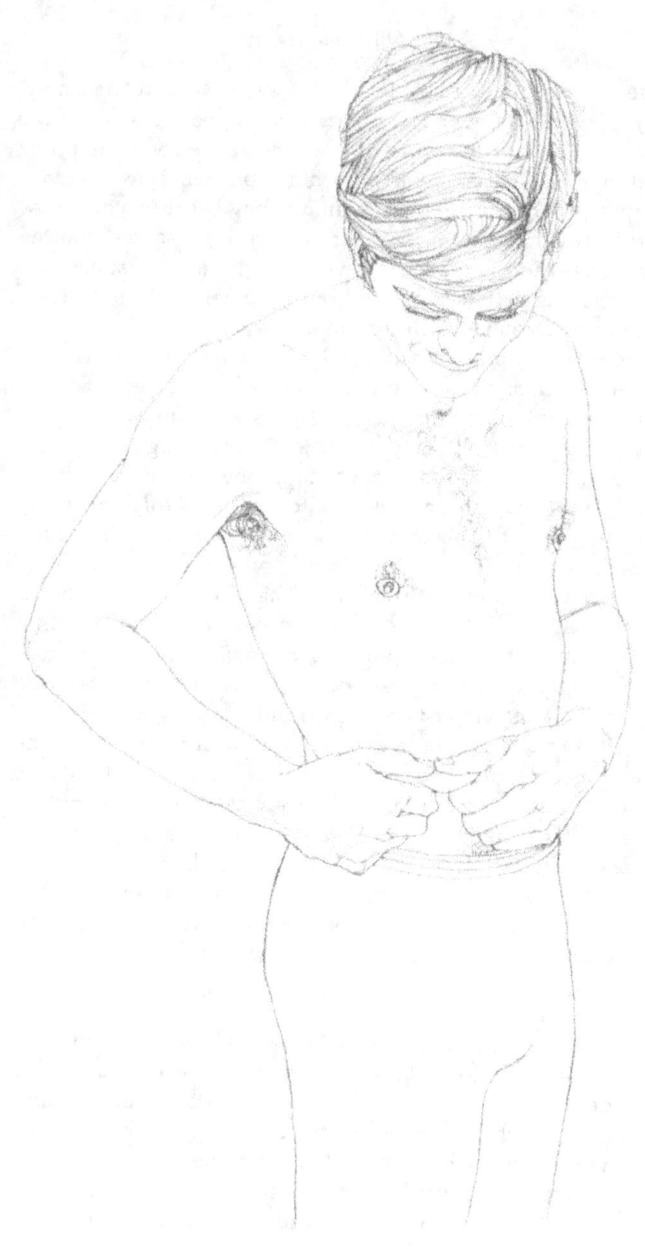

Most of the time fibrositis is a warning that something needs work. Today it may look unsightly, tomorrow you may begin to hurt.

The condition goes by several names, but by whatever name, anybody who suffers from it wishes it would go away. It won't. We call it *fibrositis;* to get rid of it, you have to make things so miserable and uncomfortable that it simply can't stay. The cure is a combination of a nutritious, controlled diet, pinching massage, and specific target exercises. The diet you will find in Chapter 12; and the massage is fully described, along with the specific exercises for target areas, on pages 174–177.

If you wonder whether or not your offending spot is fibrositis or just plain fat, pinch a roll of it in your fingers. The fibrositic area will feel exquisitely tender and it will dimple. A roll of fat pinched at the waist may look unsightly too, but it will not be tender, it will not be hard, and it won't dimple. The best example of fibrositis is the "dowager's hump" that sits right in the center of the shoulders just below the neck and is found most often on older women. The shoulders are prime targets all across their breadth, since we tighten them almost constantly and catch ourselves doing it only *after* enough damage has been done to make them react painfully. The upper arm is another target, as are the lower back, hips, thighs, knees, and the outer aspects of the lower legs and ankles.

Spot Reducing

Considerable controversy has been raised over the efficacy of spot reduction. Those taking exception to it are quite correct when they hold that you can't select a spot (like a double chin) and slim it down while ignoring everything else. No, the total program comes first. It is the "spots" that do not answer to the total program, because they are something more than merely deposits for fat that need the extra work. So if you have always had heavy thighs, "just like my mother's sister," be of good cheer. You both have the same tendency, but *you* know what to do about it. Use a total program, and *in addition*, work those "spots" until they give up.

So find out what your body measures, where the weight is coming off and where it is not. Find out where you would like some attractive muscle to add to your aura of sexuality. *Use your measurement chart every week.*

If there are other areas you wish to watch, such as the neck, the pads that sometimes form on the inner aspects of the knees, or if your ankles seem thick, add them to your list.

Arms

Measure with a relaxed arm three inches down from the armpit if you are interested in checking for fat. If you are seeking to determine the progress being made with a

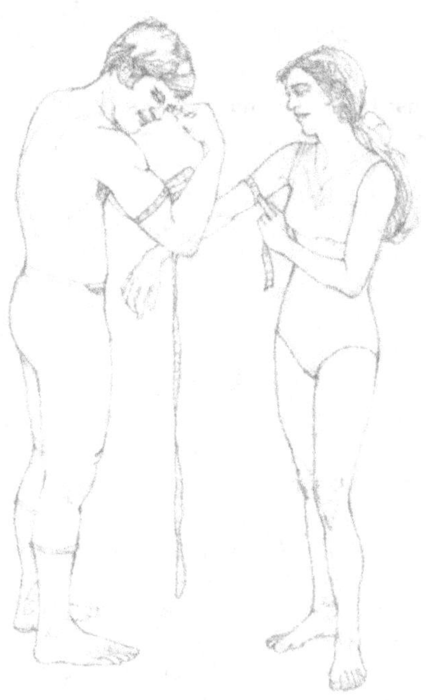

weight training program (pages 30–31), measure the same spot but with the arm contracted to "make a muscle."

Chest-Bust

Inhale fully and then let half the air out and measure across the nipples.

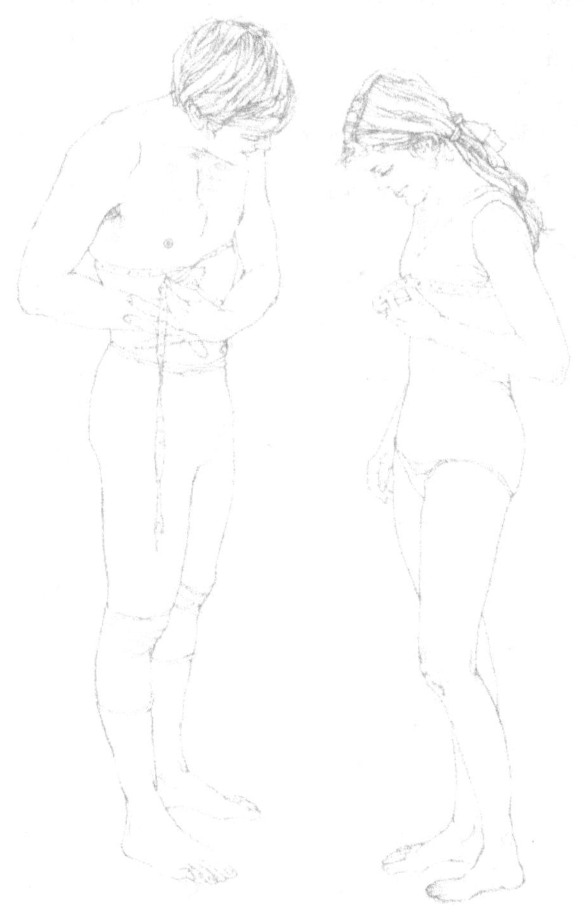

Midriff

Leave the tape measure where it is across your back but run the front under the breast to measure at the widest point of the chest (both male and female).

Waist

The waist measurement is easy enough to find, but don't pull in. You want to know the absolute truth.

Abdominals

To find the level for measuring the abdominals, lower the tape to a point just below the navel; *most* people have a slight bulge there. Also, if you pinch that bulge and

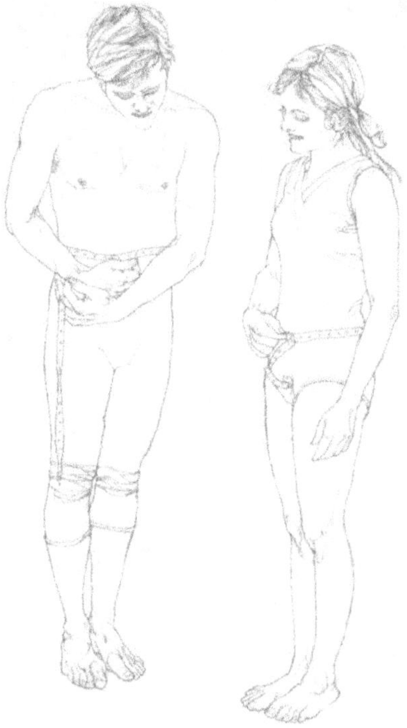

measure the roll with your fingers and find more than an inch-thick roll, you are well over the required amount.

Hips #1

Many people have a bulge *on each side* at the tops of the hips. They are sometimes called "saddlebags." Run the tape over these two bulges, being careful to see that the tape stays level.

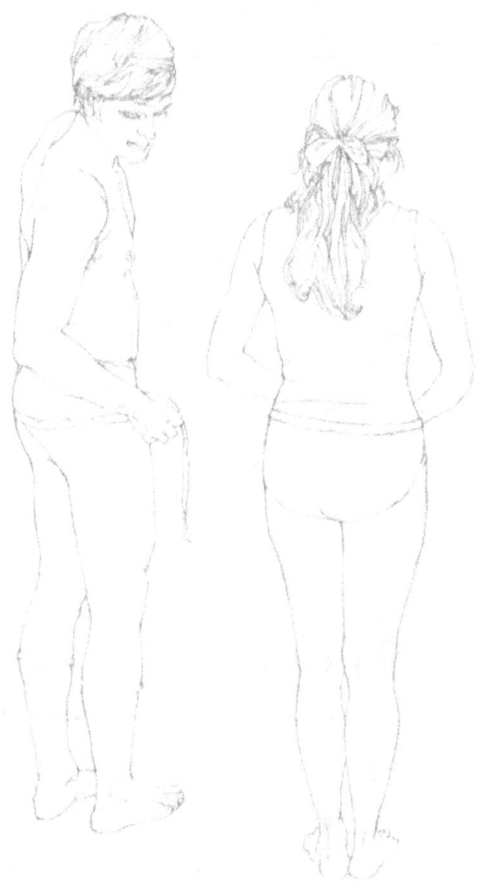

Hips # 2

Drop your tape a few inches until it surrounds the hips at their widest point.

MEASUREMENT CHART

Date					
Right arm					
Left arm					
Chest-Bust					
Midriff					
Waist					
Abdominals					
Hips #1					
Hips #2					
Right thigh					
Right knee (upper)					
Right knee (lower)					
Right calf					
Right ankle					
Left thigh					
Left knee (upper)					
Left knee (lower)					
Left calf					
Left ankle					

Thighs

To check for fat, unclothe the leg to be measured and check the thickness of the thigh at its widest point, usually about four inches down from the crotch. To check for muscle development, tighten the muscles of the thigh and measure the same place.

Above the Knee

This is a favorite tension spot and therefore subject to fatty deposits usually at the front and inside of the knees. Check about an inch above the kneecap.

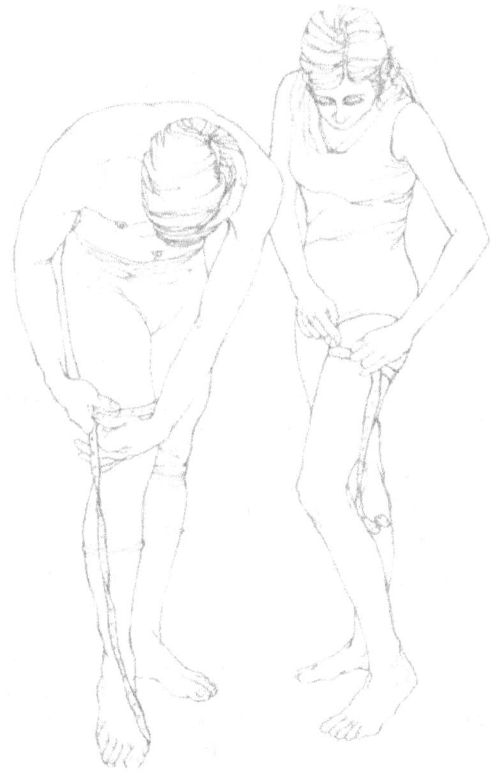

Below the Knee

This too is a favorite tension spot, and the lump usually forms on the inside of the knee and is *very* tender. Measure right below the kneecap.

The Calf

To check for fat, measure the unclothed leg at the widest and fullest part of the calf. To check for muscle development, tighten the muscle and weight the leg. You may even add a little size if you stand on the toe.

The Ankle

Most ankles (unless the area has been selected for tension) do not change very much from month to month. If they are thick, however, exercise and fibrositis (pinching) massage will certainly make a difference. If you have this problem, be sure to measure.

On the day you start your program, enter the date of your first set of measurements. One week later, at the same time of day (best before breakfast) *and without looking at the previous week's score,* enter your next set. Then compare your results. With a red pen enter the differences (plus or minus) next to the second score. Add all the *minus* inches together, and if you had any plus inches, subtract them from the minuses. Let's say you lost four inches overall (don't sneer at quarter-inch losses, they mount up), put the result, −4″, at the bottom of the third column where your comparisons are listed. Under that column you might also enter any losses in weight. The third week you will enter your measurements in the fourth column and your comparisons in red in the fifth. Let's say you had a very good week and lost five inches overall. Enter that at the bottom of the fifth column as the week's loss, but then add that week's and the one before to give you a grand total. That way you will be able to chart your progress for both the short and the long runs.

If by the third week you find that your waist and midriff have gone steadily down but your thighs haven't budged an inch, think *fibrositis* and act accordingly. If you are a woman and you find your bust measurement has increased whether you wanted it to or not, remind yourself of the fluid factor. Fluid retention comes and goes. Ignore it for the time being.

Weight

The best way to keep track of weight is daily, then it can never surprise you. Weigh in each morning without clothing and before breakfast. Keep your weight chart right there on the wall for all to see.

DAILY WEIGHT CHART
FOR ONE MONTH

Compare your weight results with your measurement results often. If the scale says you are not losing weight in spite of diet and exercise, but the measurement chart says you are losing inches, you are doing fine. Keep right on doing what you are doing. If the scale says you aren't losing and the measurement charts says you aren't losing, read the chapter on diet.

Obesity Is Spelled "Not Tonight, Josephine . . . or Joe"

Obesity is dangerous to health, an obstacle to sexuality, and a means of achieving an early end. There are virtually no very old, very fat folks.

When you are thinking of making love and of ideal partners for that lovely adventure, you won't think of a fat partner. Nope, even if *you* are fifty pounds overweight, you'll dream up a slender one, so it would be best to become one yourself if this is a problem.

Fat is deadly, and should the sexercise program you are undertaking right now result not only in a happier and more satisfying love life but also a baby (often this happens as health improves, so watch out if one isn't on the agenda), then know right now that that baby's future happiness lies in your seed. If your parents were obese, or even if one of them suffered from that distress, obesity is hidden in the blueprints your baby will use for self-development. If you or your partner is fat, so much the worse for the baby. If you do have that baby and you don't reprogram his plans during the first months of life; he will spend the rest of it fighting fat. Right from the first week, think *diet and nutrition.* If the baby is breast-fed, what the mother eats will be very important. If it is to be raised on a formula, then you'd better know all you can about the formula you are given. Read Adelle Davis' book *Let's Have Healthy Children* long before the baby arrives. That book will also help the mother with her own nutrition (and therefore the baby) during a critical time. From the very first, know that sugar is your baby's enemy, and where babies are concerned, sugar is pronounced sucrose, dextrose, and, worst of all, dextro-maltose. If your baby doesn't find out for years and years that there are such things as cookies, crackers, jelly beans, lollipops (even in the pediatrician's office!), chewing gum, soda pop, or even ice cream, then you will be able to break the pattern and reprogram the blueprint, thus saving the baby from multiplying fat cells that can and will make him miserable. There is no such thing as baby fat, puppy fat, or adolescent fat. There is only yellow, oily, parasitic, destructive fat. Banish it.

There is something else you can do if your love together brings you a baby, and that's to understand about taste. We all develop preferences for certain foods when we are very young. To our sorrow, the taste of young America is now being developed to serve the manufacturers of food products, not their own bodies, minds, or futures. Check with the chapter that covers nutrition and sex, and project that information downward into babyhood, where taste begins.

As for you, what trend is your weight taking? What did you weigh when you got out of high school? If you added as little as 1¼ pounds every three months, which is very easy to do, you will have gained twenty-five pounds one year after you get out of college. Should you marry right then and continue with your weight gain, you will have put on a grand total of fifty pounds by your fifth anniversary. If *he* started out with few fat cells and a reasonable appetite fortified by good eating habits, *he* may not have gained an ounce by that fifth, but *she* may present quite a different picture. She may have added the twenty-five since her wedding day and then complicated the increase through pregnancy. If she was cursed with hereditary fat cells and the development of unhealthy eating habits compounded by a lack of physical activity, it would be no trick at all to gain *and keep* anywhere from ten to twenty pounds with each baby.

The positions are often reversed. *She* may have had the good cells as a gift. She may also have been raised on proper food. She may have had the opportunity to become an athlete, dancer, or cheerleader, and she may have married the captain of the football team. *He,* however, may have hung up his football uniform when he graduated but kept his appetite. A football player can consume as many as six thousand calories a day with impunity. A bank teller cannot, so *he* put on those fifty pounds, which took over the space hitherto allotted to muscle. He will continue to look impressive for a while, but that's where it ends. Lovemaking is a tactile pleasure, and no matter how he looks with his clothes on, he can't *feel* like that with his clothes off. Fat isn't strong and fat isn't virile. Fat *is* dangerous, however, and on his forty-seventh birthday, just when his fourteen-year-old son needs him most, a large chunk of that fat can slip into a vital artery and kill him in ten minutes.

When you look back over the next few months with your eye on your weight chart, you will find that daily weight fluctuates and sometimes it hits a discouraging plateau. However, if the peaks and valleys and even the tableland have a downward *trend,* you can feel satisfied. The peaks too will serve a purpose—as your conscience. If you watch your diet all week and can proudly boast the loss of two pounds on Friday, that's great. But if you go all out with beer and pretzels over the weekend, you may find that you put back two and added a third. A second careful week followed by a second disastrous weekend will net an overall gain of two pounds. Such a program will make it impossible for you to fit into today's best outfit in just two months. Eight pounds is really quite a gain; keep it going for a year and it will add up to fifty-two pounds. If you took a slightly different tack, however, being careful all week and foolish only once a month, in just three months you could lose fifteen pounds, and that's a most impressive loss.

With the help of your weight chart and measurement chart, you will be able to tell just how much you lose if you exercise regularly and pay attention to your *food selection.* You will also be able to choose a program knowing full well how often you can afford to go to hell in a food cart and get away with it. You will soon know which foods have got to go, which kinds of weekends are too expensive in terms of weight, and which ones will burn up every calorie you can swallow—for example, bike touring or mountain climbing.

One thing should be remembered: when you are making love, you aren't eating. Also you can burn up as many as twenty calories a minute making love. The more love you make, the more calories you burn. The slimmer, stronger, and more vital you are, the more love you can make. Looks like an ideal reducing program and a really wonderful way to maintain the ideal weight. All you need is a partner who thinks the same way you do.

6

Sexercises

In order to improve your appearance, your physical function, and your endurance—all of which will improve the level of sexuality and general attractiveness you bring to lovemaking—you will need a program. This one has been distilled down to essentials, and all of the exercises do what is claimed for them.

You don't need every single one of them every single day. It would help if you did them all, but if that is not possible, use the sexercises this way. Before every exercise session, use the eleven warm-ups described on the next pages. These particular exercises *warm* the muscles by increasing circulation, and a warm muscle is 20 percent more efficient than a cold one (also safer from injury). If you can take time out to do them before engaging in sports, especially sports like tennis, you may avoid muscle damage and will certainly improve your game.

After you have done your warm-ups, move on to each of the exercise sections—standing, kneeling, prone, supine—and do at least two in each section. Do all of the pelvic tilts, however, and all of the flexibility exercises. Once a week, for really tremendous results, go through the whole set.

Music

Americans will do *anything* to music. They love rhythm, and they have rhythm. If you can manage to work to music provided by records or tapes, you can select the kind of music that pleases you and lifts you off the floor. That makes exercise fun and easy. When two or more people work together, music helps them stay together and gives the work form. Just as it's easier to march together to a good beat, it's easier to exercise together to a good beat.

Clothing

Remember that you are using these exercises to achieve a higher level of sexuality, and appearance *does* count, even to your own subconscious. Flo Ziegfeld always dressed his beautiful showgirls in the real thing, whatever the real thing was supposed to be, from imported Spanish lace to silver fox furs. He said that when a woman is dressed for the part, she becomes the part. The same thing is true for men, and that has been the reason through the ages for all those stunning uniforms. Wear something appropriate, and your old baggy sweat pants are not appropriate, especially if you've been sweating in them. A nightgown isn't a good idea; hard physical work will play hob with its fragility, and besides, it will get in the way. Bermuda shorts and slacks bind, and foot coverings of any kind are definitely out. A leotard moves easily with the female body. Either dancer's tights or form-fitting trunks are fine for the male body: as soon as you have the chest you want, leave the top in the drawer.

Warm-ups

7. Swim

Increases circulation; loosens tight shoulders, arms, upper back, and waist; stretches hamstrings

Stand with legs wide apart and knees held stiff. Lean straight forward from the hips and employ an overarm (crawl) swim stroke, reaching as far forward as possible so that on each stroke your arms straighten and *stretch.* Do eight.

Twist your body to the left, keeping your legs as they were. Use the same swim motion, but emphasize the stroke with the right arm; this will stretch all along the right side of the body. Do eight, then swing to the right, emphasizing the left-arm stroke. End with eight more, straight forward.

8. Waist Twists—Up and Down

Separates upper and lower halves of torso; improves flexibility and slims waist; loosens shoulders and upper back, works chest

Stand with legs wide apart and knees stiff. Raise arms, with elbows bent, to shoulder level, hands in front of chest. Pull the right elbow hard right and back. Follow with the rest of the upper body. Then pull hard left with the left elbow. The rest of the torso follows along to the left. Let the leading elbow do the pulling. Alternate for eight.

Now, lean forward from the hips. Keeping the legs and hips still, and without moving the head, use the arms and hands in a punching motion, letting the shoulders follow the fists. Do eight.

Then stand straight. Alternate *waist twists—up and down* for three sets.

9. Lateral Single Knee Bend

Strengthens thigh muscles (quadriceps) and knees; stretches crotch and thigh muscles

Start this exercise with only a slight knee bend, and as your legs become stronger, drop lower and lower until you are at full knee bend. Stand with legs spread wide and feet turned slightly outward. Spread arms for balance. Bend the left knee and lean the upper body slightly to the left. Look down at the bent knee and be sure you cannot see your toes under the outside. If you can, you are pronating (rolling over onto the inside of your foot). Cover the toes with the knee. Straighten the knee and stand for two counts as you tighten abdominals, gluteals (seat muscles), thighs, calves, and foot muscles; then bend to the other side. Alternate eight times.

As you get stronger, add two steps to the exercise. Drop lower in your bend until you can go all the way down and come back up and then hold for two counts as you contract.

Then use this exercise as though there were a roof over your head, and you cannot stand straight after the knee bend but must instead move from side to side with your head at the level of the first bend.

10. Overhead Reach

Stretches shoulders and sides of torso

Stand with feet well apart and knees stiff. Start with both hands along the sides of your thighs and then raise your right arm straight overhead. Slide your left hand slowly down your leg. This will bend your body to the left and bring your right arm into the correct position for the exercise. Holding the bend to the side, draw your right hand back to cover your right ear, and then stretch it out straight again to the side. Do four to each side to make up one set; then do a second set.

11. Alternate Toe Raises ►

Increases foot circulation, strength, and flexibility; strengthens and improves shape of calf muscles

Stand with weight evenly distributed on both feet, which are parallel, about two inches apart. Keeping the toes and the ball of the foot tight to the floor, raise one heel as high as possible, trying to increase the arch by pushing the instep forward. *Don't let the ball of the foot leave the floor.* Replace that heel on the floor and raise the other one. Alternate feet sixteen times.

When your balance is secure, bring your feet closer together and try raising one heel as you lower the other, so that the feet pass each other, one on its way up and the other on its way down. Do sixteen.

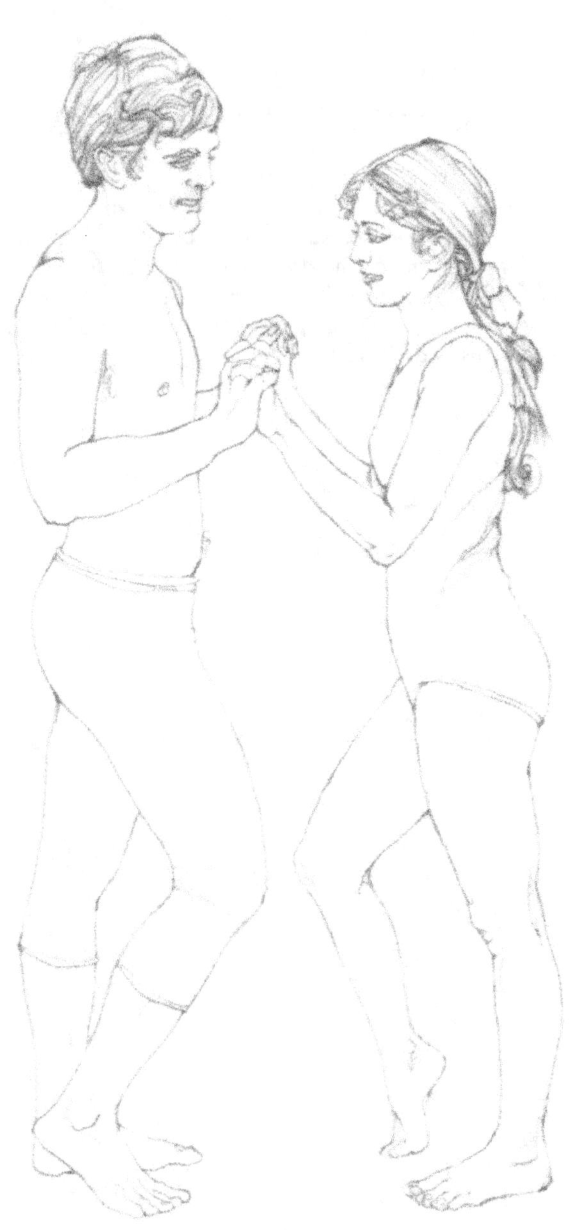

12. Snap and Stretch

Strengthens the shoulders, arms, and upper back; stretches the pectorals (chest muscles)

Stand with feet apart and raise bent arms to shoulder level, with hands in front of the chest and overlapping each other by at least six inches. On count number one, maintaining the arms at shoulder level, *snap* both bent elbows back. On the count of two, return to the starting position with the hands overlapping. On the count of three, fling both arms wide in full stretch. On four, return to the

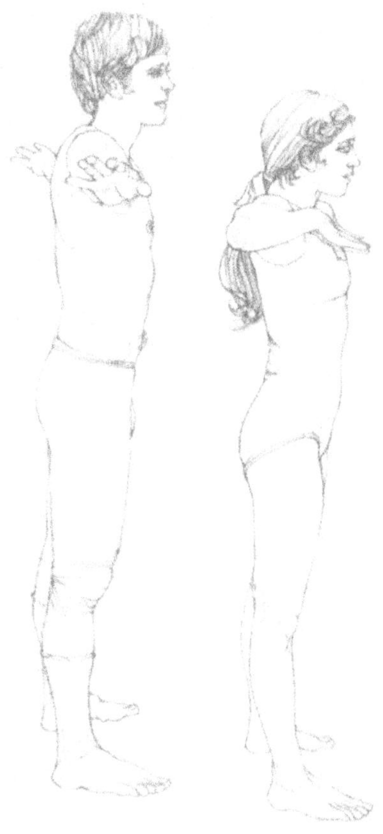

overlap. Each time you overlap, try for further reach and alternate the hands. Do eight snap-and-stretch exercises.

13. Toe Raises with Pelvic Tilt

Strengthens feet, calves, quadriceps, abdominals, and gluteals

Start with feet and knees tight together. Contract seat and abdominal muscles, and as you rise to your toes, tilt your pelvis under and press the knees forward. The level of your head should remain constant. Do eight.

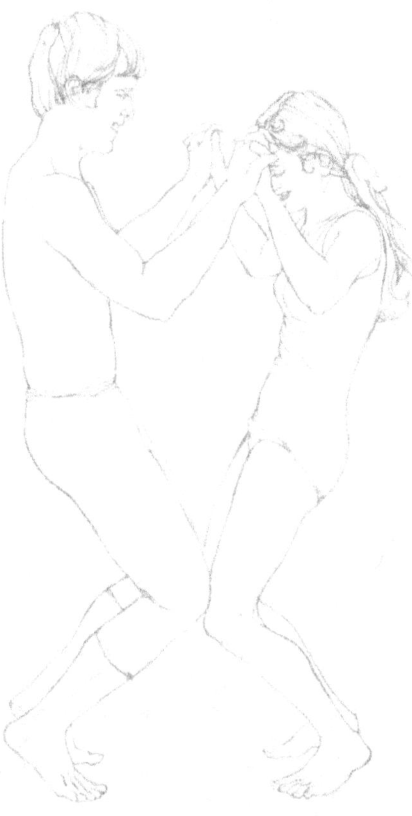

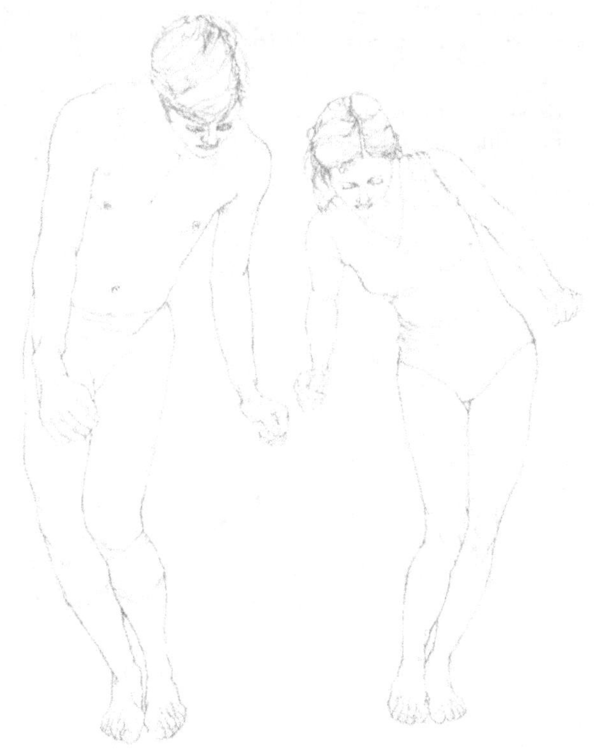

15. Bent-Knee Foot Roll

Improves foot circulation, strength, and flexibility; strengthens quadriceps and abdominals

Start with feet close together, arms hanging free. Bend both knees, and holding the bend, roll both feet onto their right sides. Then, without straightening your legs or raising the level of your head, roll both feet over onto their left sides. The farther you push your knees in the direction of the roll, the better the roll will be. Do sixteen.

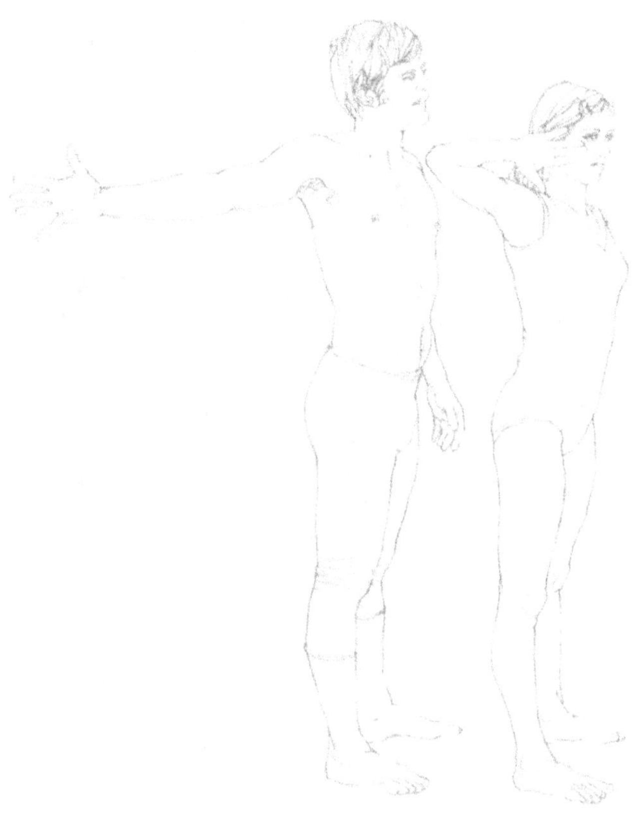

14. Back Stroke

Loosens shoulders; stretches pectorals; strengthens upper back

Stand with feet together, arms hanging loosely at your sides. Place the back of your left hand next to your left cheek, and without twisting your shoulders, press your left elbow back as far as possible. Holding that position, bring the rest of your arm to full back-stretch. Keeping the arm stretched, complete the circle and bring it to your side as you place the back of your right hand to your right cheek. Alternate sides eight times.

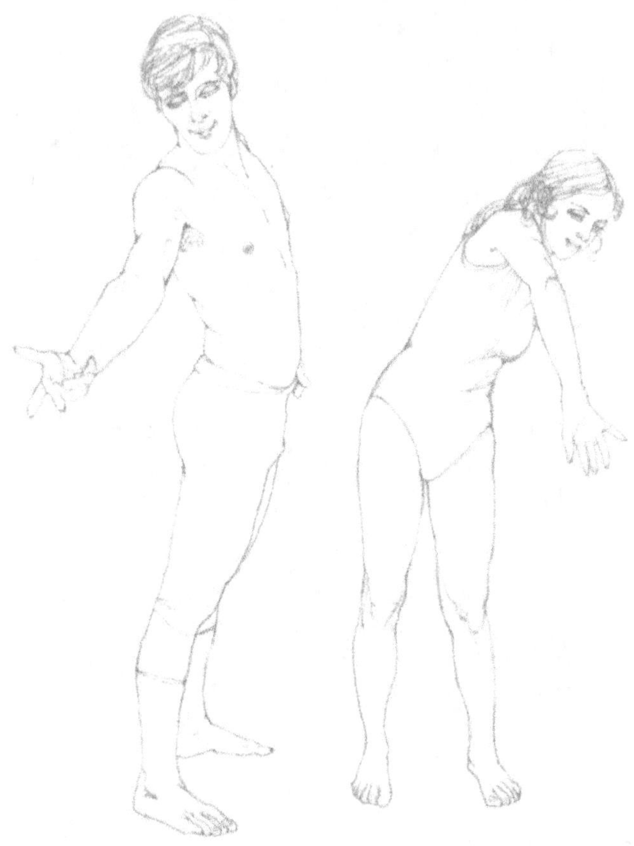

16. Shoulder Rotation

Loosens shoulders; stretches upper back and pectorals; strengthens and stretches upper arms

Stand with feet slightly apart for balance. Lean forward slightly as you twist your right arm inward and back as far as possible. Try to make your thumb point straight up. Next, twist the arm outward and back as you stand straight. Try to twist far enough so that your little finger points straight up. Do four such twists with each arm to make up a set. Do three sets.

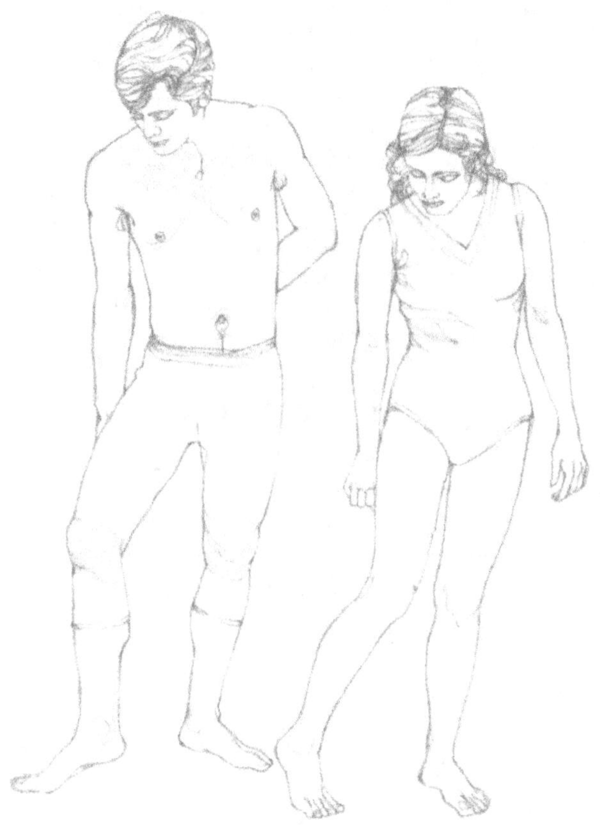

17. Hip Rotation

Improves both strength and flexibility of thighs, crotch, and hips

Stand with your full weight on your left foot and rotate the right leg inward, twisting the foot in until you can touch the floor with your little toe. Then rotate outward, trying to make the foot twist as far to the side as possible. *Both knees remain slightly bent* for the full exercise. Do eight to a side to make up a set. Do three sets.

You have probably already noticed that you have never been asked to do any one exercise more than a few times, and also that you have not been required to use the same muscles very long, but have constantly moved from arms to torso to feet. This is the secret of exercising both vigorously and long without stiffness. Allow one area of the body to dispose of the products of fatigue, such as lactic acid, while you continue to keep moving by utilizing another part of the body.

Get through as many of these warm-up exercises as you can in the course of one pop record, usually about three minutes. If you were unable to complete the series, use the same record again as you finish them.

Exercises on All Fours

Choose two of these each time you do your program, but not always the same two.

18. Walkout

Strengthens arms, chest, shoulders, abdominals, and back; stretches hamstrings

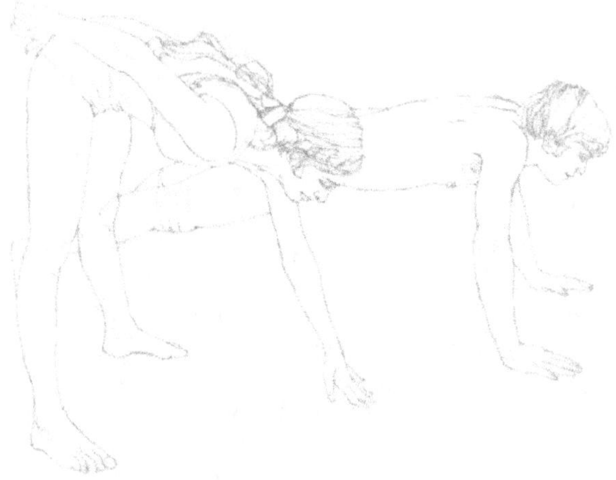

Stand with legs well spread (the farther the spread, the easier the exercise); turn feet *slightly* outward and let arms hang loose at your sides. Lean forward from the hips, and without bending your knees, walk forward with your hands for four steps, starting on the left hand. You should be at full stretch on the fourth hand-step. Allow your body to arch downward on that fourth count. Push back up, taking two steps for the return and two counts to get back up to the straight-standing starting position. On the second walkout lead with the right hand. Do eight. (You may have to start with two, or even one.)

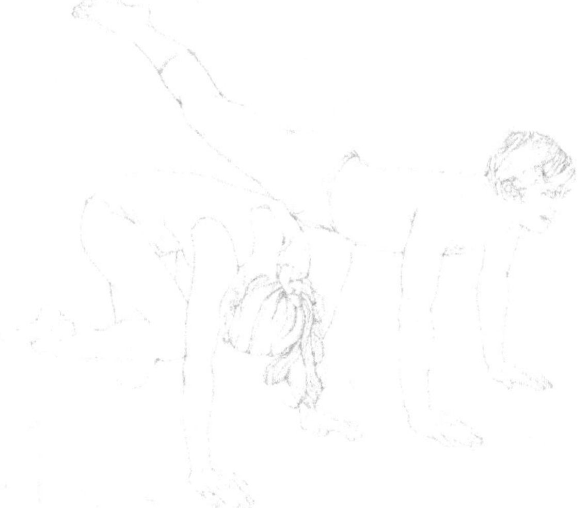

19. Knee-to-Nose Kick

Stretches back and abdominals; strengthens gluteals; slims hips

Start on hands and knees and keep arms stiff and straight. Bring the left knee as close to your nose as possible as you duck your head to meet it. Then carry that same left leg back and up as high as you can lift it. At the same time, raise your head high. Do four with each leg to make up a set. Do two sets.

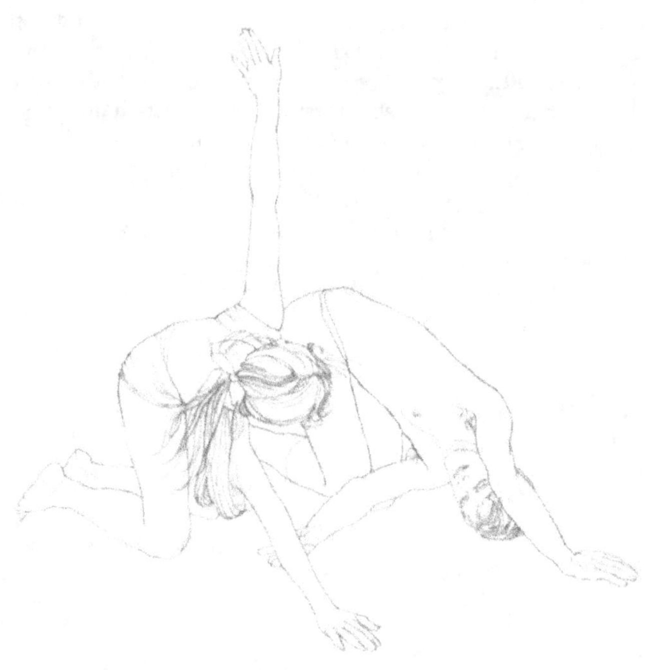

20. Thread Needle from Knees

Loosens and strengthens shoulders and torso muscles; stretches pectorals and upper back

Start on hands and knees, and twisting the upper body, reach through the space between your right arm and right leg with your left arm. Let your head almost touch the floor as you reach. Then twist back and fling the straight left arm upward as you turn your head to watch it. Do four, then change arms to do four more to the other side. Those comprise a set. Do two sets.

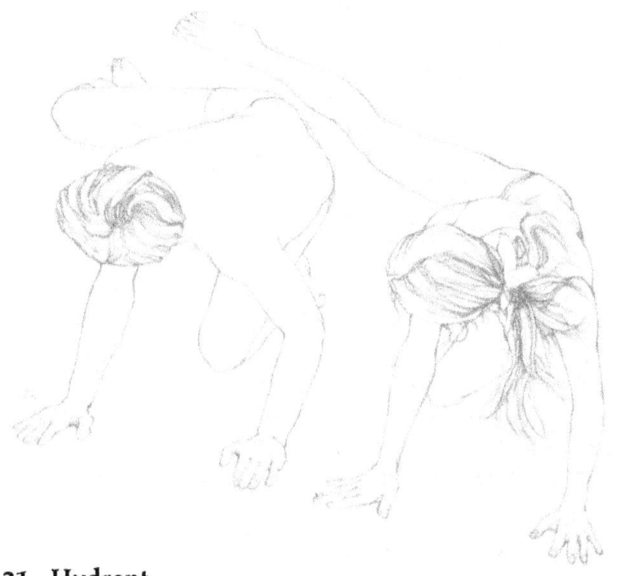

21. Hydrant

Slims the hips, especially the lumps high on the outsides, known as "saddlebags"; strengthens legs and hips

Start on all fours, and keeping the right knee in the bent position, raise it to the side. Without changing the level of the raised knee, straighten the leg until it is at right angles to the body. Bring the leg back to the lifted bent-knee position and stretch it back and up as you did in exercise 19. This will relieve the pressure on the muscles and make it possible to do another. Do four to each side.

22. Peanut Push

Strengthens arms, back, and chest; improves flexibility in abdominals and back

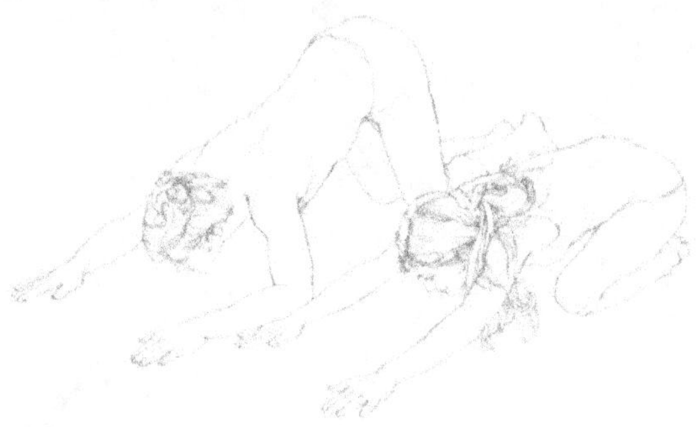

Start on hands and knees with seat resting on heels, chest on knees, and arms stretched full length in front. Pretend you are pushing a peanut across the floor with your chin. That means you keep your chin low but your head up as best you can. Go forward as far as you can,

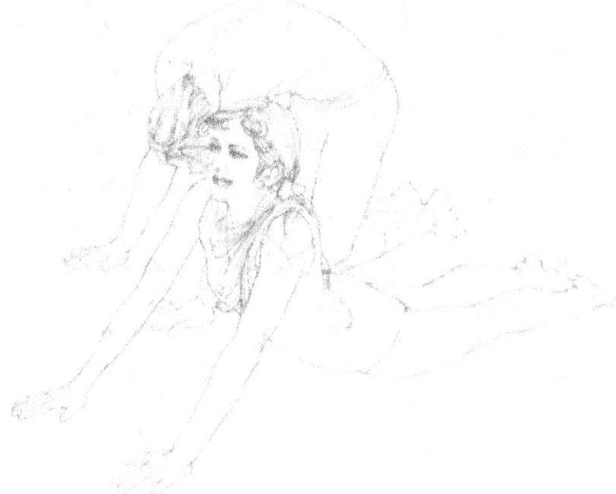

and when you are at full body stretch, push up into an *arched-down* position. Then, dropping your head and lifting your back into an *arched-up* position, push back to sit again on your heels. Start with two and work up to eight.

23. Thread Needle Standing

Strengthens arms, shoulders, upper back, and chest; stretches chest muscles and upper back

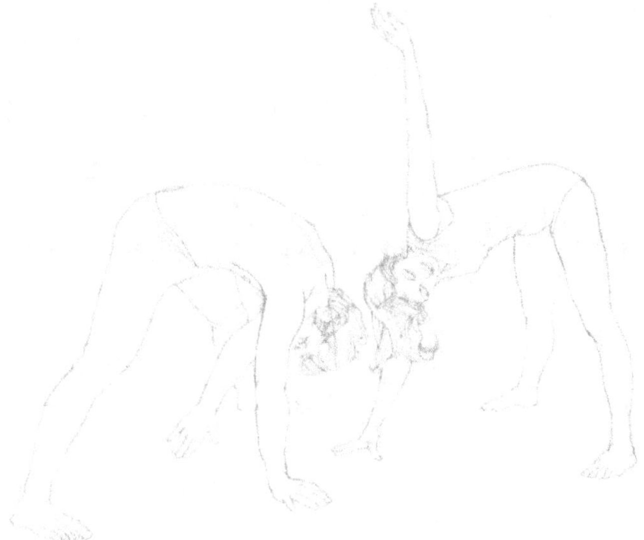

Spread legs wide, weight resting on both feet and the right arm. Reach under the body and to the right with the left arm, then draw it back and fling it straight upward, following it with your eyes. Repeat four times and then do the same with the other arm.

24. Crib Rock

Strengthens arms and chest muscles; stretches abdominals; improves back flexibility

Start on hands and knees, seat resting on heels, chest on knees. Reach as far forward as possible with straight arms. Press the weight forward onto your arms so that your

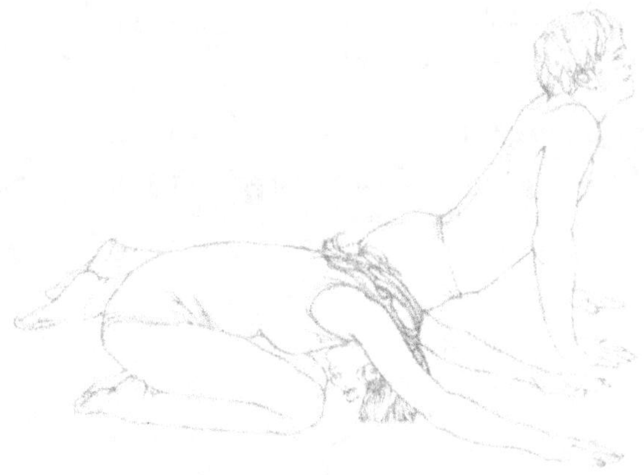

body is at full stretch with back *arched down.* Your head should be up. Return to the compact position, sitting on your heels. Do eight.

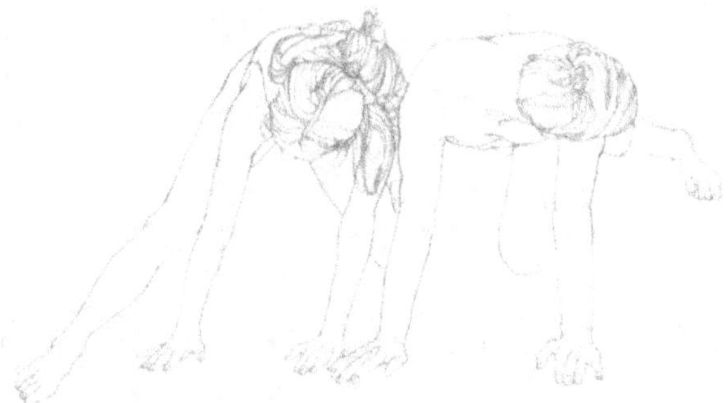

25. Back Crossover

Strengthens and slims hips; stretches sides of torso

Start on hands and knees. Straightening the right leg, swing it across in back *over* the left leg. Turn head and eyes to find it as the foot comes across. Next, keeping the leg stiff, swing it all the way around to the right, trying to set the foot down on a line or ahead of the right hand. Do four swings with each leg to make up a set. Do two sets.

Exercises in the Prone Position

Start with one in the series and slowly add the others as strength improves. This series strengthens (and slims where necessary) upper and lower back, hips, arms, and legs; it also stretches the chest muscles.

26. Arm and Leg Lifts

Lie prone, (face-down) with legs straight and arms stretched straight above the head. Lift one arm from the floor and put it down, then the other. Do not roll your chest from side to side. Alternate arms, doing eight to a side, then go on to the leg lifts.

Raise first one leg and lower it, then raise the other and lower it. Alternate eight times to a side, trying to get each leg as high as possible. Now combine the arm and leg lifts.

Raise the right arm and the left leg at the same time,

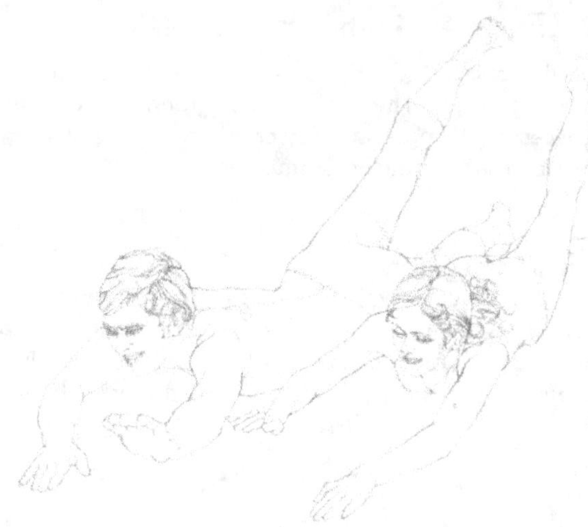

and then lower. Raise the left arm and right leg simultaneously and lower. Alternate sixteen times.

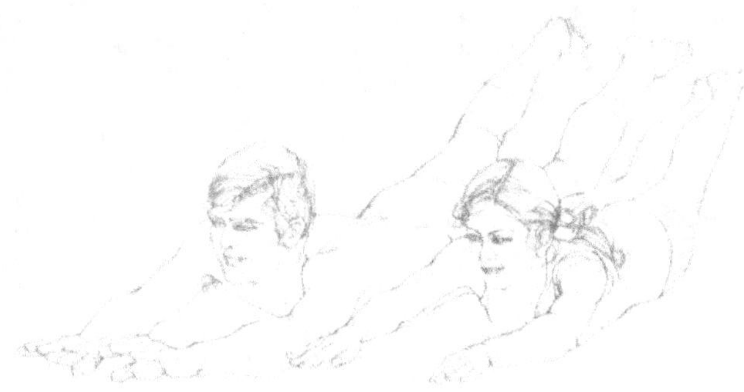

27. Double Arm and Leg Lifts

Lie prone and lift both arms at the same time; lower. Do eight.

Lift both legs at the same time and then lower. Do eight.

Lift both arms and both legs at the same time; lower. Do eight.

28. Back Crossover

Lie prone, with hands placed on the floor on a level with your shoulders, elbows *slightly* bent. Spread legs wide. Keeping your hands in place, lift the right leg and swing it back and over the left leg. Bend your knee and arch your back as you try to bring the right foot to touch the left hand. *The hand does not move.* Replace the leg in its starting position, and swing the left across, endeavoring to touch the right hand with the left foot. Do four at the start, but work up to eight.

Side-Lying Exercises

Choose two different ones for each session.

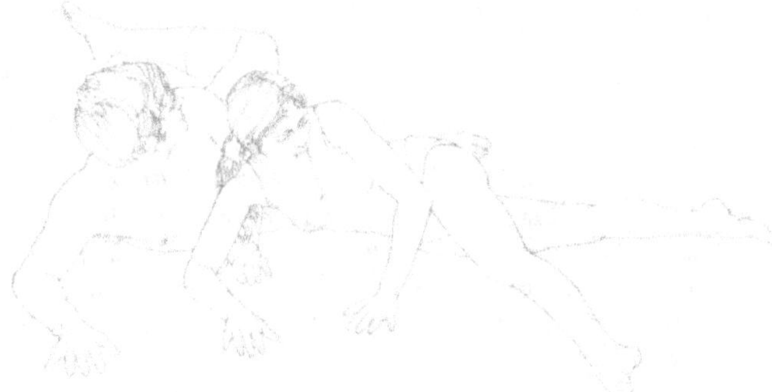

29. Crossover

Strengthens lower back, abdominals, hips, and legs; stretches abdominals and crotch

Lie on your right side with body weight resting on the right elbow. Place the left hand on the floor in front for better control. Swing the straight left leg forward to touch the floor at right angles to the other leg. Next, swing the same leg backward, allowing it to bend as you press for distance. Do eight on the right side and then eight on the left.

30. Leg Lifts

Stretches crotch and hamstrings; strengthens legs

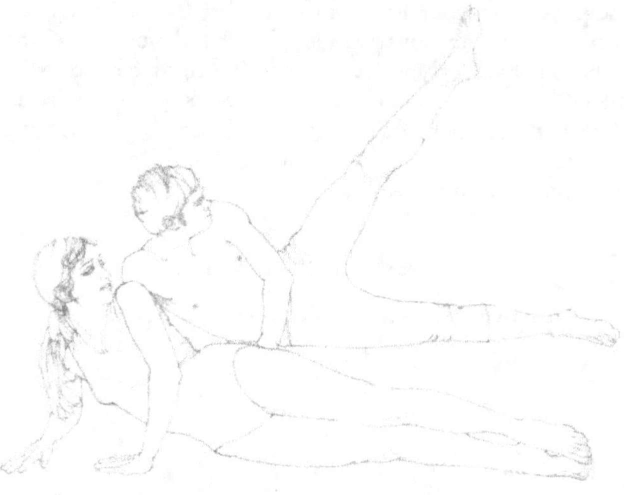

Lie on your right side, resting on your right arm, which is bent. Place the left hand on the floor in front for good control. Raise the left leg as high as possible without rolling back onto your hip. Do four, roll over onto the left side, and repeat. Do four to each side for a set. Do three sets.

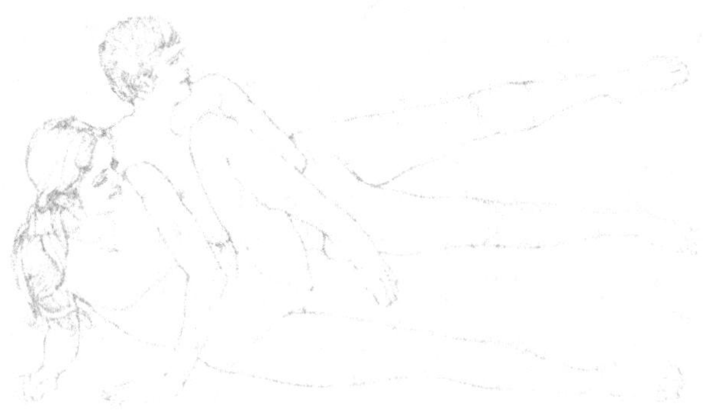

Again on your right side, bring your left knee in the bent position as close to your left shoulder as possible. Press it *behind* your left arm. Then extend the leg down to a point where it is directly above the right, with about a foot of distance between them. Bend and extend eight times to a side.

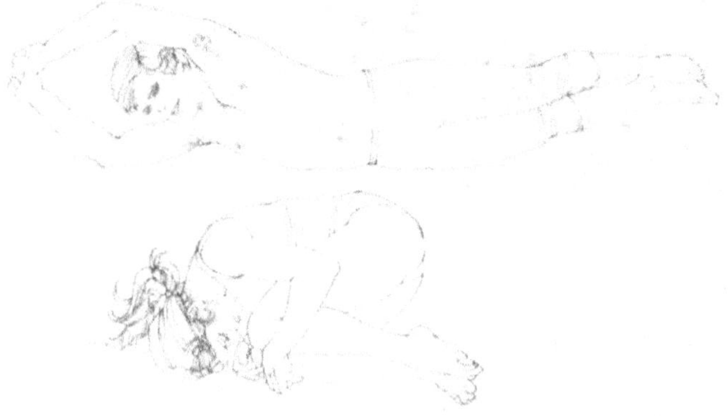

31. Curl, Stretch, and Roll

Stretches back and abdominals; strengthens abdominals

Curl into a ball while lying on your right side. Stretch your body to full length, with arms overhead and back arched. When you roll to the other side, do so by raising your legs, shoulders, head, and arms *slightly*. The roll is made on your seat. As you roll past the center position, curl to the other side. Then stretch, arch, and roll back to the starting position. Do eight.

Sitting and Supine Exercises

Choose two for each session.

32. Sit-ups with Arm Throw

Strengthens the abdominals and removes the "pot" (Note: The only time you do sit-ups with straight legs is when your arms are free to either throw or reach forward as an assist. This is not because you can't sit up without help; it is because when the arms are behind the head, it puts a strain on the lower back—a prime cause of back pain.) ➤

Lie supine, with knees bent and arms stretched full length overhead and resting on the floor. Swing your arms forward as you round your back and drop your chin to your chest. Roll up to a sitting position and reach forward as far as possible. Then roll slowly down again to the starting position, trying to feel each separate segment of your spine as it touches the floor. When your back is flat on the floor, reach overhead and repeat. Do four.

33. Flagpole ➤

Strengthens abdominals; stretches back and hamstrings

Lie supine at full stretch, and as you raise one leg straight up, reach for the raised ankle with both hands. In the beginning, you may have to walk your hands up your leg rather than simply reach. Leave your leg in the vertical position and lie back to rest on the floor. Repeat the reach four times to each side.

34. Drop-to-the-Side Toe-Touch ➤

Strengthens abdominals; stretches back, pectorals, hamstrings

Sit with legs spread wide, and twisting the upper body to the right, place your right hand as far to the right on the floor behind you as you can reach. Drop the upper body toward the floor, catching it on both hands and resting the side of your head on the floor. Push back up and reach forward to touch your toes as you swoop around to repeat the exercise to the left side. Do eight.

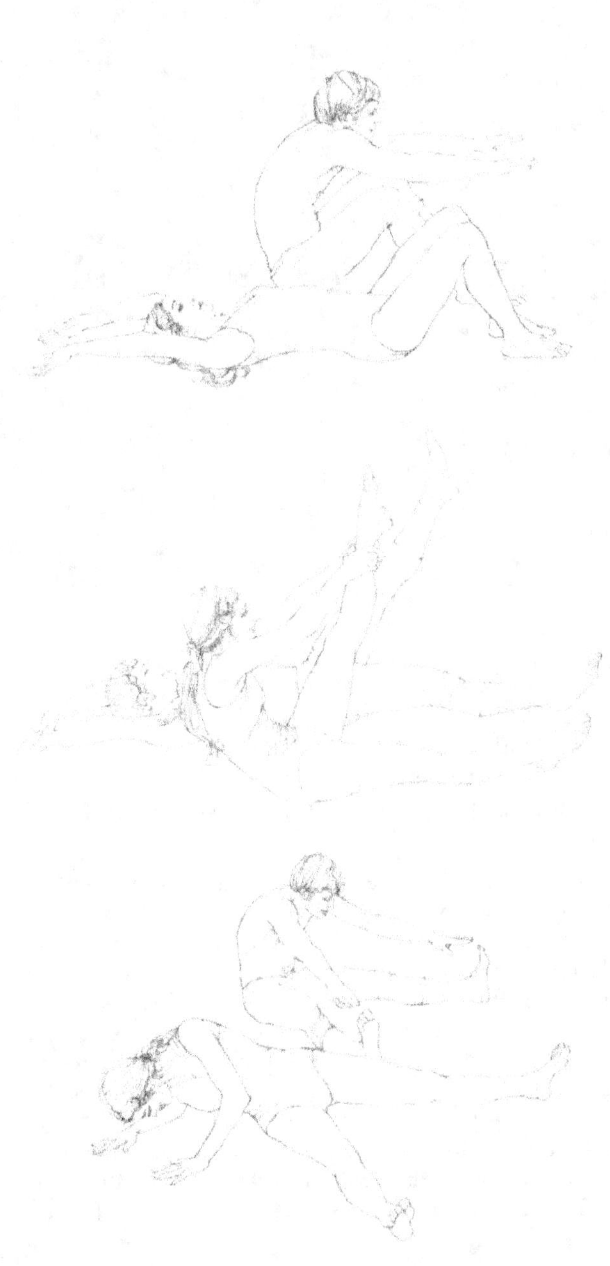

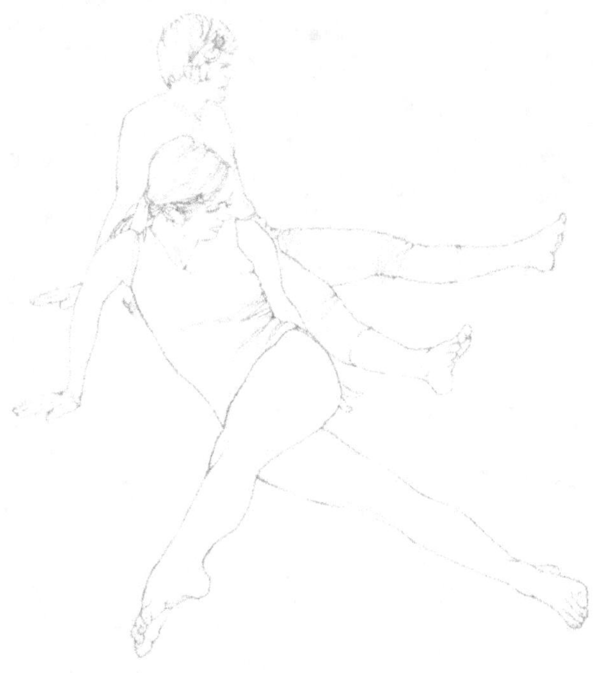

35. Thigh Rotations

Strengthens and stretches thigh muscles; strengthens abdominals

Sit with legs spread wide as you lean back on straight arms. Turn the toes of the left foot inward as far as you can. This will rotate the thigh muscles inward as well. Lift the foot with the leg straight and carry it across over the right leg and touch the floor with the big toe. Keeping the leg in the same position as for the toe-touch, turn the foot outward, which will rotate the thigh muscles. Carry the straight leg with turned-out foot all the way back to the spread position and touch down with the little toe. Keep the leg in the same position as you rotate the foot inward to repeat the exercise. Do four to each side to make up a set. Do three sets.

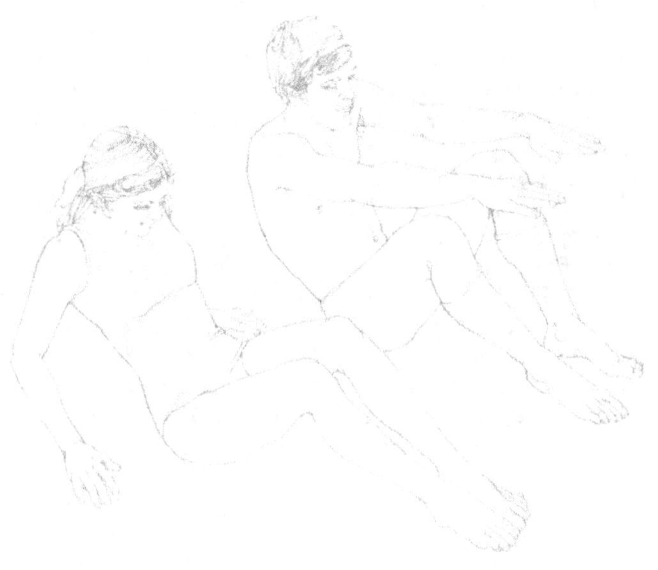

36. Foot Bounces

Strengthens abdominals and thigh muscles

Sit with knees bent and hands resting on the floor just back of your seat. Using a good fast beat, do the following series:

(a) Bounce feet up and down straight in front of you eight times.

(b) Bounce feet together, but from side to side, eight times.

(c) Bounce feet in scissors fashion, one forward and one back, eight times.

(d) Bounce feet as in (a) and add the hands banging on the floor to the same beat. Eight times.

(e) Keep the foot bounce going and hit the floor with your hands on each of three foot bounces. On the fourth bounce, throw hands in the air. Do sixteen.

The Pelvis

Making love is a physical act—and a very physical one, at that. The average *healthy* person will drive the normal pulse beat of 72 up to 150 beats a minute, which is the same as that of a top athlete during maximum effort. Back muscles, buttocks, abdominals, and thighs are worked harder, faster, and longer than even in the most demanding sports. Remember, even the miler quits after four-plus minutes! The foregoing exercise program was designed to build strength and improve flexibility in every part of the body leading to the center. The center, or *pelvis,* is the main instrument, but only an instrument. By itself, it isn't much—rather like the all-important wheels of your car. The wheels get you where you want to go, all right, but without the engine, they are without movement. Until fairly recently, there was almost nothing in our culture that

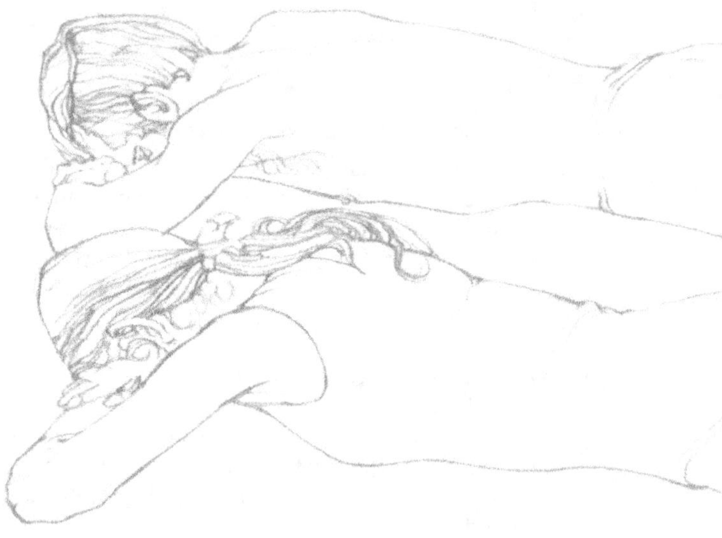

developed pelvis power. And unless you are an aficionado of rock or African-influenced dance, you still may be deprived when it comes to pelvis power. But that can be remedied. Let's take it from the very beginning, even if you think you already know it all.

37. Gluteal Set, or Pelvic Tilt—Prone

The gluteals are the muscles in the buttocks; it is their forward drive, as well as the contractions of the abdominals, that brings two bodies together. If your seat looks soft and mushy, or if it answers to a separate rhythm of its own when you jump up and down, instead of being all of a piece with the rest of you, your gluteals are weak and therefore not up to the expert job you should expect. If the gluteals are soft, they won't drive. So you start right there.

Lie prone on the floor with your head resting on

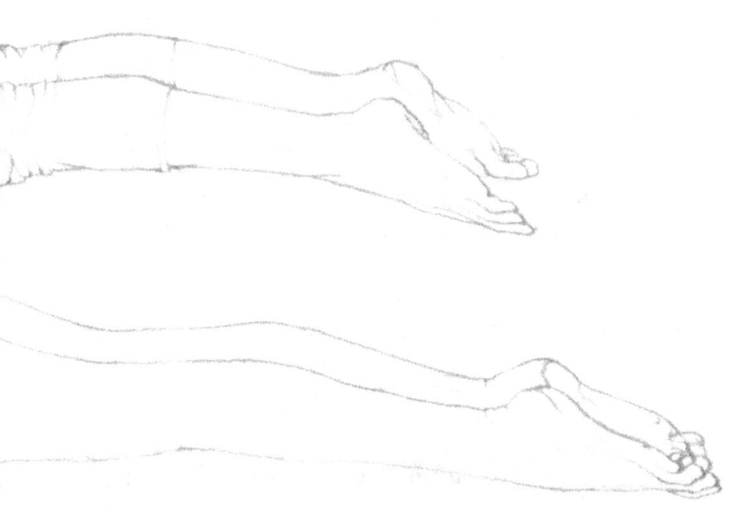

your arms. Tighten your seat (or gluteals) by pinching the buttocks tight together. Hold the contraction for a slow count of five and then relax. That relaxation is very important. To be efficient, a muscle must not only be able to contract. It must also be able to give up contraction completely. Do this part of the exercise three or four times, giving special attention to the relaxation. If you find it hard to let go completely, roll both heels outward and it will help. Then add the next step, abdominal contraction. Start by tightening the buttocks and then pull in the abdominals. As you tighten one against the other, the pelvis will tip under as it should when making love. Slide your hands under your abdomen. There should be about one inch of space there. If there isn't, you are either not pulling in hard enough or not tilting under hard enough. Or maybe there's just too much of you in the abdominal area. In that case, use the fibrositis massage (page 174) even on the too-opulent abdominals, and do exercise 1 every chance you get. Don't forget to consult the chapter on dieting for sexuality. Start with three gluteal sets and work up to ten.

Gluteal sets should be learned in the prone position, but once you know how, use them all the time and everywhere. While you wait in line, tighten. As you go up and down in elevators, tighten. When the meeting or the class is dull, and even while you stand waiting for the light to change, tighten. You need never again feel you are wasting time. Just tighten and think about how you are going to use your ever-improving skill.

38. Pelvic Tilt—Supine

The pelvis must be strong enough to thrust downward as in exercise 37, but it must also be strong enough to thrust upward, and this is much harder, because the powerful gluteals cannot help quite so much and the abdominals have to do most of the work. The longer you can maintain the natural backward and forward motion in an exercise, the better you can control it when it comes to the real thing. Lie on your back with knees bent and feet about eighteen inches apart. Keeping your shoulders and seat tight to the floor, arch your back slightly. Then forcing your spine downward,

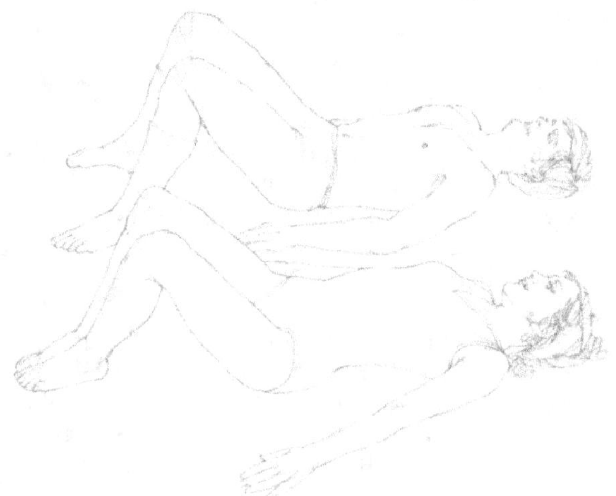

tilt your pelvis under. There are muscles inside the pelvis that need exercise too. They are called the levators, and they can be worked by consciously tightening the sphincters. In case you haven't run across that word before, a sphincter is a ringlike muscle that surrounds a passage or entrance to the body, the ones you exercise to keep you from becoming socially unacceptable. Tighten everything you can find in your pelvic area, and hold for a slow count of five. Then relax completely. Repeat the series of slight arch, spine down contraction-hold, and complete relaxation five times.

39. Sphincter Series—Mostly for Women

After you have tightened *everything* for exercise 38, you will be able to locate the sphincter muscles consciously and without difficulty, which doesn't mean they are doing all they can do for you. Some people are born with the ability to tighten and relax the pelvic muscles many times in rapid succession and to achieve contractions that are of considerable strength. Not everyone is so lucky. Others have to work at it.

Sit in a chair and contract all those muscles in the pelvis, and then let go. You will soon see how easy it is to contract and how hard to let go, but it is the letting go that determines how often you will be able to contract, how fast, and how completely. Here is another exercise to fill what might be called wasted time. Tighten and relax slowly and evenly four times. If you cannot relax your contraction completely, push a little, which may help to inform those muscles as to what is expected; this will pattern them for you.

Next, divide the contraction and relaxation into four steps each. Imagine each contraction to be the length of four inches and contract "one inch" at a time. The fourth and last will be strong and easy, the first tentative, the second stronger, and the third hard to keep separate from the fourth. To make them even in strength will take work. Reversing the procedure from the hard fourth contraction to the first "inch" of relaxation isn't difficult, but to separate the second and third "inches" from the others will be. You may have to *push* to get the final "inch," that is, to achieve complete relaxation. Practice.

Finally, the fourth contraction and the first "inch" of relaxing are key movements in making love. Tighten your abdominals to lift the weight from the pelvis and tighten to the "fourth inch." Let go for just the "first inch" of relaxation and tighten again. Use music to set up a rhythm to which you try to adhere. Contract-relax on every beat for eight counts, then relax, even push loose for the next eight counts. Four or five sets of eight will feel as tiring as many knee bends would feel to thigh muscles, but, like the thigh muscles, the sphincters and levators will improve, and you will achieve more for your effort than just stronger muscles.

The man who learns to control these muscles can increase the frequency of orgasm by a technique known as seminal retention. By tightening these muscles just as orgasm is about to begin, the amount of semen discharged at ejaculation is decreased, and he can retain enough for an extra sexual episode and climax. This is something worth the price of admission all by itself, but there is no need to elaborate on this point. I've told you what you need to know.

40. Seat Lift *(see pages 94–95)*

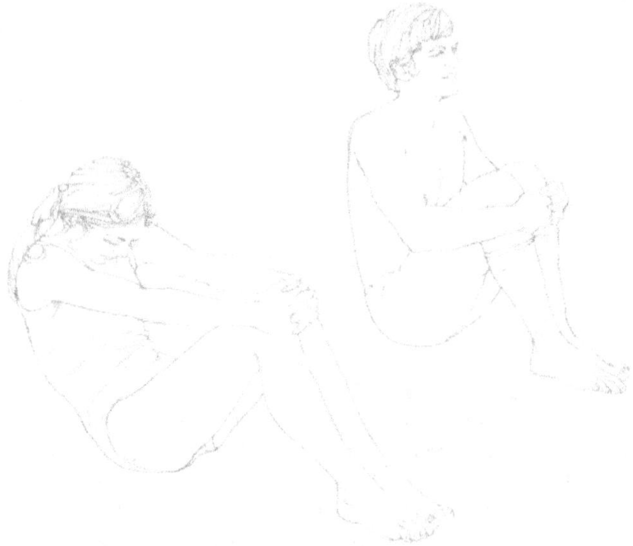

41. Pelvic Tilt—Sitting

It should be noted that very little goes on in life without the benefit of the pelvis. In addition to increasing the skill and pleasure of lovemaking, every exercise for the pelvis improves posture, guards against backache, prevents fatigue, reconditions after childbirth,

(continued on page 96)

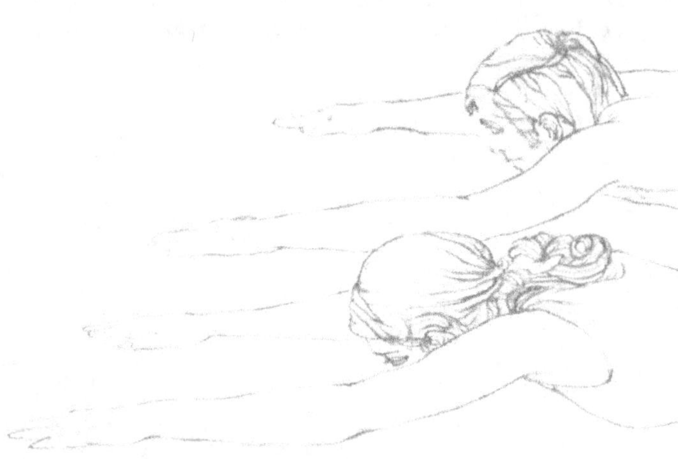

40. Seat Lift

This is an exercise for people who already have strong, limber backs. The value of this exercise to the male is in endowing him with the back strength and flexibility he needs for making love in the traditional position. For the female, it provides both strength and flexibility for the prone position, either as active or passive partner. If passive, which would happen in the prone position under the male, levator strength for action *inside* the pelvis is a must.

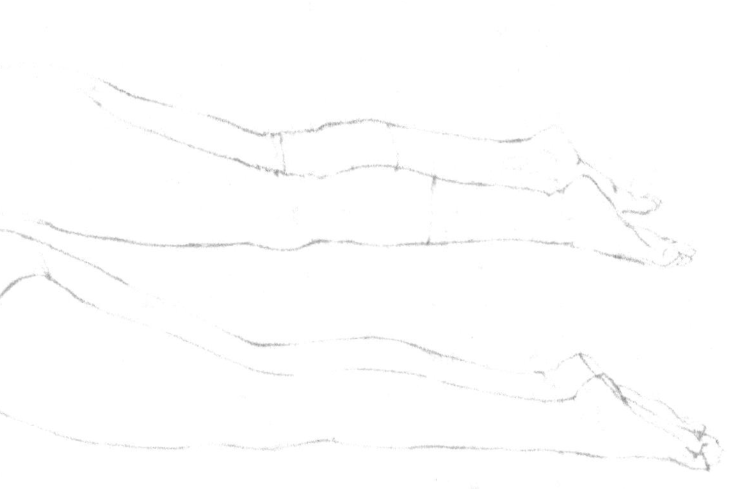

It is not only lovers, but also people with flat backs who need this exercise, as well as all the other pelvic tilts. Dancers, gymnasts, and horseback riders will find this exercise easy. Football players will not.

We teach seat lift to children by telling them to "paint" the floor under their chests with glue and then place their chests down in that glue and stay stuck. Then we tell them to raise their seats in the air and hold for four slow counts and then lower. Alternate this exercise with exercise 37, six times.

improves form in any sport, and certainly affords a better figure for both men and women.

Sit on the floor and clasp your hands in front of bent knees. If you have one of those prominent tailbones that aches at the movies, the pressure will interfere with your work. Take a bath towel and fold it in half the long way. Then take the two farthest ends and fold them into the middle. Fold the edges into the middle once more and you will have a cushion with a space running down the center. Sit on it so the tailbone rests in the center, and there will be no painful friction. This can be used for sit-ups as well.

Holding your hands in front of your knees, lean back with your head down and spine rounded backward. Tighten your abdominals and round your shoulders as much as possible. Find the levators and tighten them too as you hold for a slow count of four. Then straighten your back, throw your shoulders back, and lift your head. Release the abdominals and levators. If you can arch your back, so much the better. Hold for four counts, and repeat the lean-back. Do eight.

42. Pelvic Tilt—Kneeling

This exercise not only calls for "tilting," "tightening," and "relaxing" the gluteals, abdominals, and levators; it also demands thigh strength and instep stretch. You *should* be able to lay your insteps flat on the floor, and age has nothing to do with the fact that yours may look like Japanese garden bridges. Such inflexibility means that you have tightened your ankles and foot muscles when under pressure, and you have finally foreshortened the muscles. Sooner or later you will hear from those mishandled muscles, and if you merely "walk old" long before your time, that will be the least of it. One way to lengthen them is to get down on your hands and knees. Lift your weight from your knees, shifting it to your hands and the tops of your insteps for two or three seconds. Lower and repeat. If your foot goes into a cramp, wiggle your toes and it will stop. Do at least four such lifts every time you exercise (more after a bad day). It will help if, after they stretch a bit, you will bounce your weight downward in short easy bounces. For the present, until your insteps are stretched, you will have to do your kneeling tilts with a rolled hand towel under your insteps.

Start on your knees as you sit back on your heels. Push your seat way out and try to arch your back. Without raising the level of your head more than a couple of inches, move your seat under and tilt your pelvis. Tighten the abdominals and levators in the forward position. Relax them as you return to the back-arch position. Do four of these kneeling tilts at the start. Work up to eight.

43. Pelvic Tilt on All Fours—Cat Back

Start on all fours with straight arms, and keep the arms straight all through the exercise. First, arch your back upward like an angry cat. Tighten levators, abdominals, and gluteals; hold for four counts. Be sure your head hangs downward and your neck is relaxed.

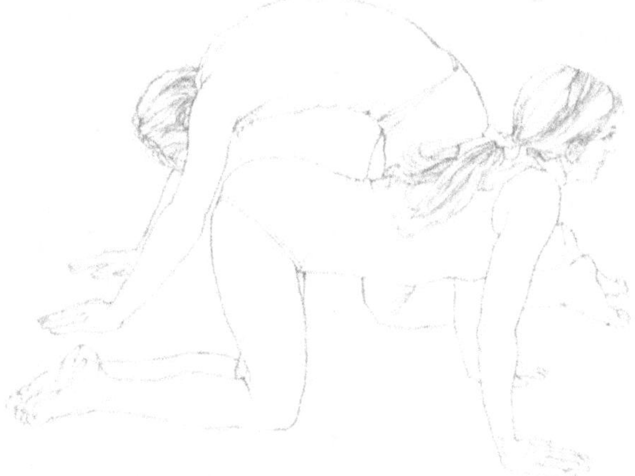

Next, allow your back to sag like that of a tired old horse. Relax abdominals, levators, and gluteals and raise your head high. Keep arms straight. Rest for a second or two and repeat. Do eight.

44. Pelvic Tilt—Standing

Stand with feet apart and knees slightly bent. Rest your hands just above your knees and thrust your seat out as you arch your back. Keep your head up. If someone were to swat that exposed seat with a canoe paddle and it was against the rules to run, jump, let go of your knees, or straighten your legs, what would you do? You would tighten your unprotected posterior into a hard knot and tip the pelvis under, hard. Use all the knowledge you have acquired and pull in *everything*. Hold for a count of four and then take the starting position for another four counts. Do four of these, counting four in each position. As soon as you find you can make the transition from back-arch position to pelvic-tilt position smoothly, saying tilt-two-three-four, back-two-three-four, double your time. Take two counts to tilt and two counts to arch back. Do sixteen. Much later, cut the time to one beat for each movement. Again, do sixteen at a time.

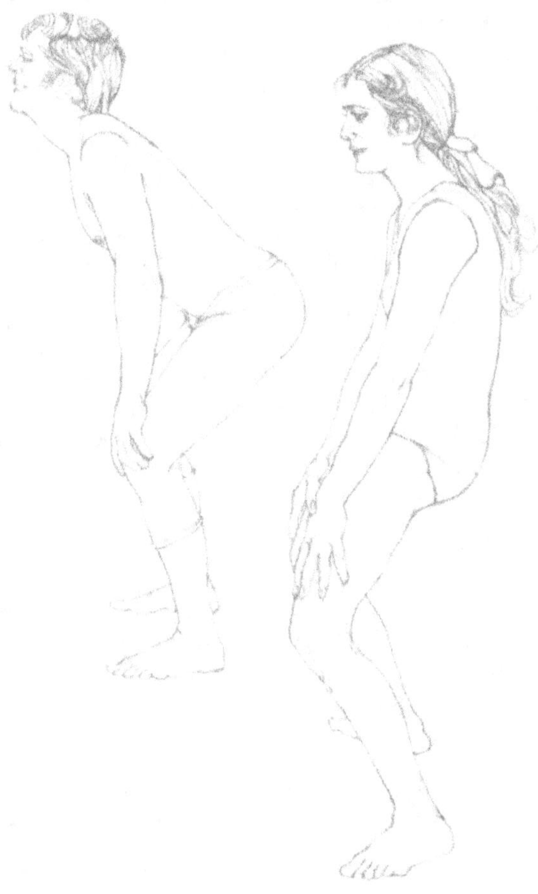

45. Pelvic Walk Series

Keeping feet flat on the floor, walk across the room, taking eight steps, with your body held in the starting position for exercise 44. At the end of those eight steps, take eight more with the pelvis tucked under. Alternate in this way several times, and when you find you can make the transition even while moving, cut down to four steps for each movement, still later to two counts for each. When the inevitable comes and you are down to one step for each movement, you will find that the forward tilt will always happen over the same foot. Cross the room that way, and then cross back, tilting forward over the other foot.

You will be getting into the big time, so to speak, when you can bang out two tilts to each step. At the start, use a slow beat for this. African drum rhythms are best. Step forward, and as you take your weight on your foot, tilt, and tilt again. Bring the other foot forward and repeat. Do this exercise whenever you can. It's a great way to improve pelvic action. The new dances have much to offer in this area, especially the currently popular belly dancing. The only trouble with that particular form of dance is the mistaken idea that it is for women only. Men can easily omit the come-hither arm movements and retain the important pelvic action.

46. Hip Swing—Arm Reach

The basic hip-swing movement is made by shifting the pelvic area, or hips, from side to side while keeping the upper body still. This is an excellent exercise for any sport that requires that the upper half of the torso move separately from the lower (skiing, riding, or gymnastics, for example).

Stand with feet apart and legs held stiff. Extend both arms to the sides, and without moving the upper body, shift the hips from side to side. The break will occur at the waist.

Next, bend both knees slightly and swing again. The knees will follow the direction of the swing. When that comes easily, do as you did in the pelvic walk at the end of the series and try to swing twice to the right and then twice to the left, taking most of your weight first on the right foot for two and then the left for two.

There are many combinations, all of them useful. Try doing the double hip swing to the right and then to the left four times, and then walking forward four steps, doing a double forward tilt on each foot. After you can tilt up a storm, you will suddenly discover that today's music (most of it) has been written to encourage just such action.

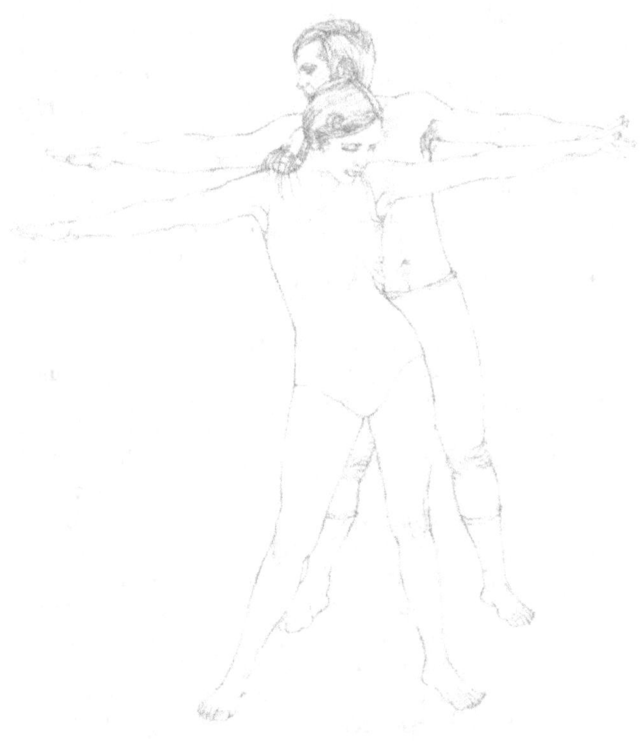

Sex and Flexibility

The most sensuous-looking animal we know of is the cat. She stretches constantly, moves with lightning speed when she wants to, and lies utterly relaxed when she chooses. Cats are beautifully balanced, and they have the ultimate in coordination, because they are both strong and flexible. Think of a cat and then think of the most tense individual you know, perhaps yourself. Do you ever stretch like a cat? When you lie down to rest, are you immediately relaxed like a cat? When you arise, are you rested and do you cross the room with a fluid motion? When you've been sitting in your car for a couple of hours, how do you walk when you stand up? When you have worked long hours at your desk, how do your shoulders feel?

The rate at which we lose our flexibility determines the rate at which we will age. Those who are flexible have many advantages in terms of coordination, freedom from stiffness and pain, appearance in movement, and the ability to get the most from rest. And certainly they are to be envied when it comes to making love.

Flexibility is the degree to which a muscle can give up tension, and is determined by personality, way of life, the degree of tension to which we have been subjected daily, and what we use for physical release.

While we are still very young, we begin unconsciously to select our own particular areas for tensing whenever under stress. Since parents have a great deal to do with our tensions, we can thank them for at least the start of what one day may cause us misery and is capable of ruining our lives. That statement was not made lightly or in order to point a finger at parents, who, heaven knows, get plenty of that as it is. It is made so that *you* will know how to handle the tensions of *your* children. No parents can prevent tension from exacting some toll from their children, but the wise parent can combat tension by seeing to it that the children have plenty of physical outlets that exercise every part of the body. In years to come, those children would be able to say, "My tension must be in my shoulders, because they are stiff and painful. I imagine swimming would help."

With children, however, one cannot tell just where the target area is unless they hunch their shoulders or show other clear physical signs of tension. The answer to that problem is to present a variety of physical outlets, ones that release tension in general. That means vigorous forms of exercise that spread their benefits.

The observable signs of constant tensing—round shoulders; aching backs, jaws, shoulders and necks; thickened thighs and ankles; heavy hips and arms; the dowager's hump; and an inability to turn far enough to see behind you to park your car—those come *after* the damage has been done. They can be mended if you want to mend them, but only if you know how and are willing to work for it.

Here are a few good reasons for making such an effort. The ability to mold one's body close into another's depends to a great extent on flexibility. The ability to make love for a long winter's afternoon, or whenever, depends not on strength and endurance alone but on flexibility as well. The "how-to" books present a vast array of positions, most of which any flexible person making love with another flexible person already knows all about. Flexibility not only *permits* variety, it *suggests* it. Now, the question is, how does one acquire it?

Muscles that are tensed over and over again, without benefit of relieving stretch, become foreshortened. When the shortening becomes constant, the bony framework responds to the pull, and the posture anomalies become apparent. Since we sit in chairs rather than cross-legged on the ground, we don't notice the narrowed range of the crotch or low back stretch, but we *feel* it soon enough, usually while making love. Sad to relate, the phrase "If you've never had it you won't miss it" also applies to freedom from tightness, strain, and unnatural pull in muscles. If you've never been free of it, you have no idea how wonderfully your body would move and feel.

Do the following flexibility exercises every day, preceded by a few warm-ups. One thing that is certain for all of us is that none of us will escape tension, even when the only stresses are noise, heat, cold, and crowding. If the stress is more deadly, as, for example, that caused by worry, deadlines, unhappiness, fear, or anger, you will need protection. The protection is here.

(Note: Be sure to warm up before doing these exercises.)

47. Widespread Leg Stretch

Primarily for the hamstrings, but does include the lower back

Sit with legs spread wide and grasp the left ankle with your left hand and just under the calf with the right hand. Using your arms to pull your body down toward your leg, keep your head up and pretend you are trying to put your chin on your big toe. Bounce your upper body downward in eight easy pulls and then straighten.

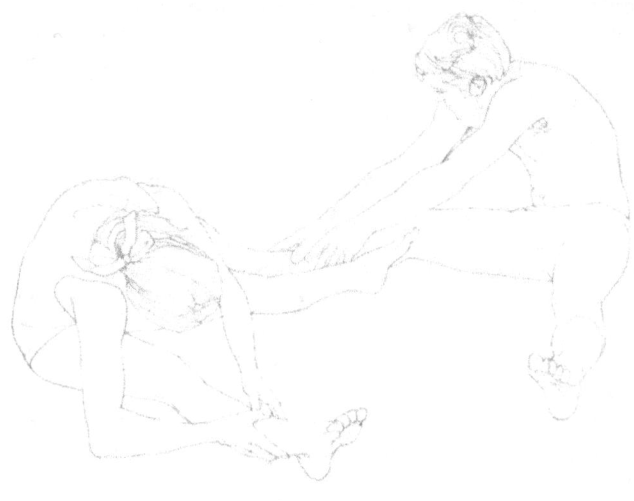

Drop to the other side and repeat the eight bounces. That makes up a set. Do three sets.

Holding your legs the same way, try to pull your left ear down to touch your left knee for eight bounces, and then do the same on the right. Do three sets. Be sure to keep your knees absolutely straight and your feet turned *slightly* outward.

48. Heel Pull

Hamstring exercise used for combating too much sitting

Rest back on your left elbow as you lie on your left side. Bend your right knee and place your right hand *inside* the right leg under the right heel. Holding the heel, straighten the leg. Bend and straighten four times and then roll to the other side and repeat. That makes up one set. Do two. (If straightening the leg while holding the heel is out of the question, grasp the ankle. Just make sure you exert plenty of pressure to the resistant hamstrings.)

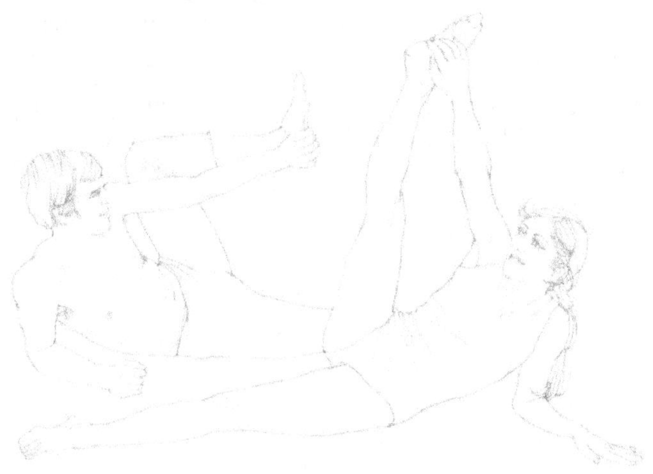

49. Side-Drop with Toe-Touch ►

Hamstrings, chest, and shoulders

Sit with legs together or slightly apart and twist the upper body to the right. Try to place your right hand behind you as far to the right as possible. Drop down on both hands so that your chest is almost touching the floor. Swing back up and lean forward to touch your toes. Continue the swing, and drop down to the left. Do eight sets.

50. Crotch Stretch ►

Sit with feet drawn up, sole to sole, close to your body. Grasp your ankles and rest your elbows on your thighs.

With the help of your partner, press down with your elbows in a steady pressure. Close your eyes and try to find where the muscles are resisting. If you want to see how well this concentration works, have someone hold a ruler by your knee while you press down without thinking, but with eyes open. Then close your eyes and think away that tight spot. The knees will drop stil' farther. Hold your press for at least ten seconds and then release *slowly*. If you let go suddenly, you will suffer discomfort. Do six.

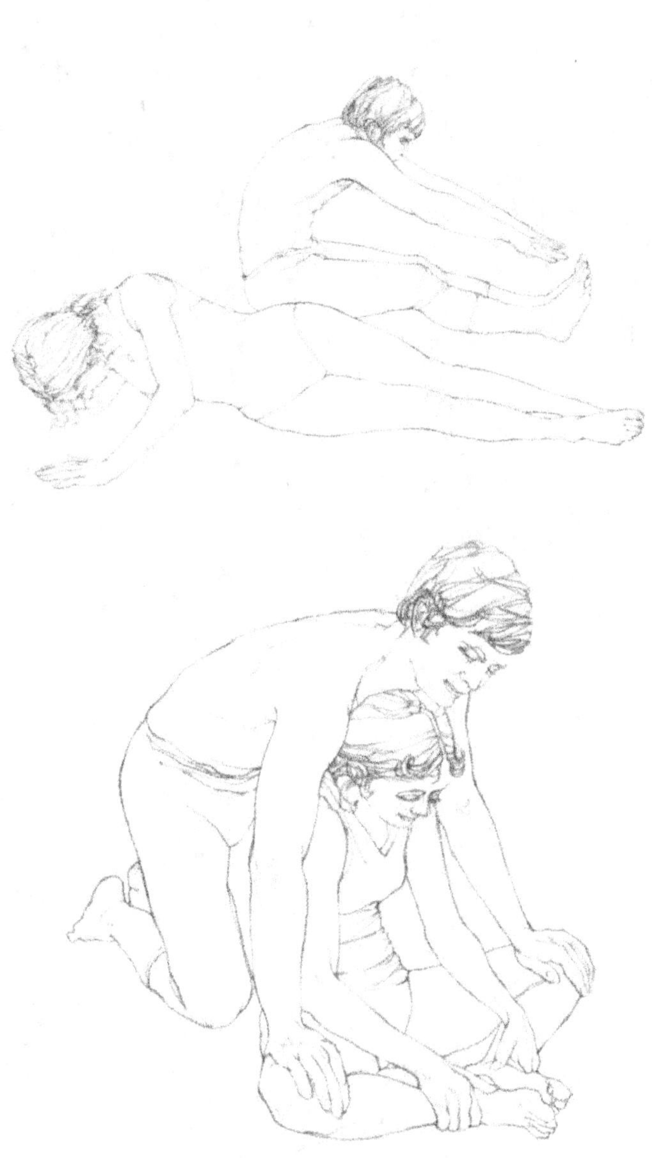

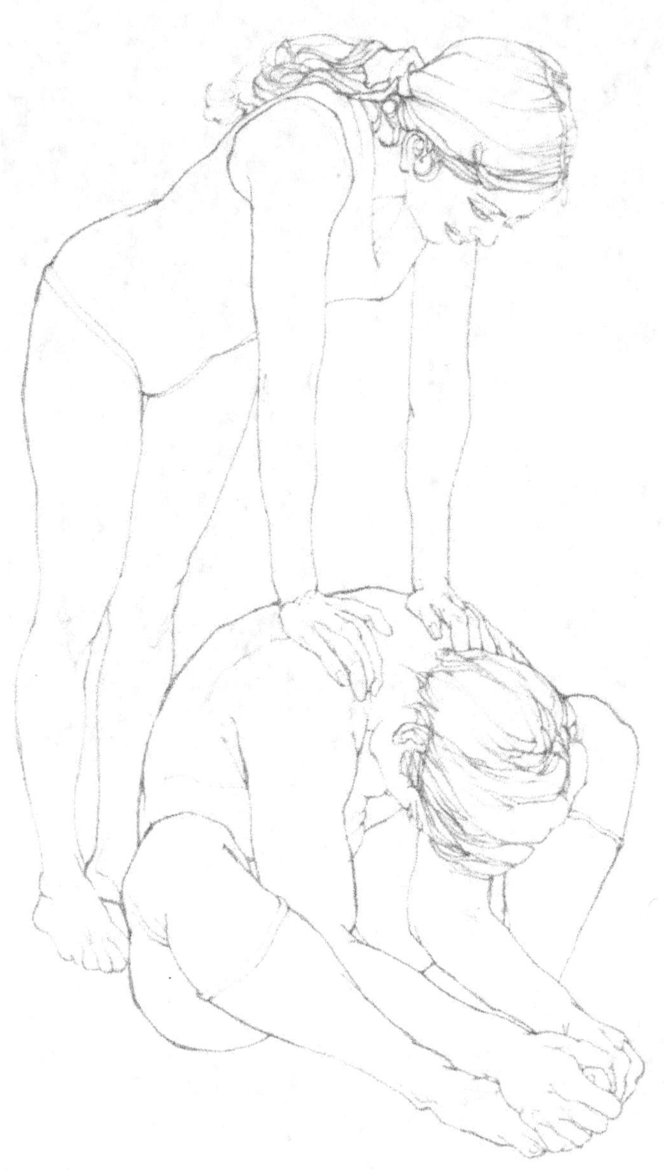

◄

51. Low Back Stretch

Sitting with feet drawn up close to the body and placed sole-to-sole, grasp the ankles and with the help of your partner try to pull your head down to touch your feet. Use the same eyes-closed concentration at the peak of your pull to find the tight places and release them. If you will have someone watch your lower back, even if you are so flexible that you can touch your feet with your head, he will notice the muscles give up tension and stretch even farther. Hold your pulls for at least ten seconds and release. Do six.

Dual Exercises

People rarely like to exercise alone, and in the case of sexercises it is unlikely that they would have to. But, so far, you could have done the exercises with or without a partner. Now you will need one.

52. Rotated Bent-Knee Sit-up

Abdominal strength and waist slimming

One partner lies on the floor with knees bent and feet placed fairly well apart, hands clasped behind his head. The other kneels in front and applies plenty of pressure to both ankles as an anchor.

Roll over onto the right shoulder and maintain the twisted attitude as you lift your upper body toward the

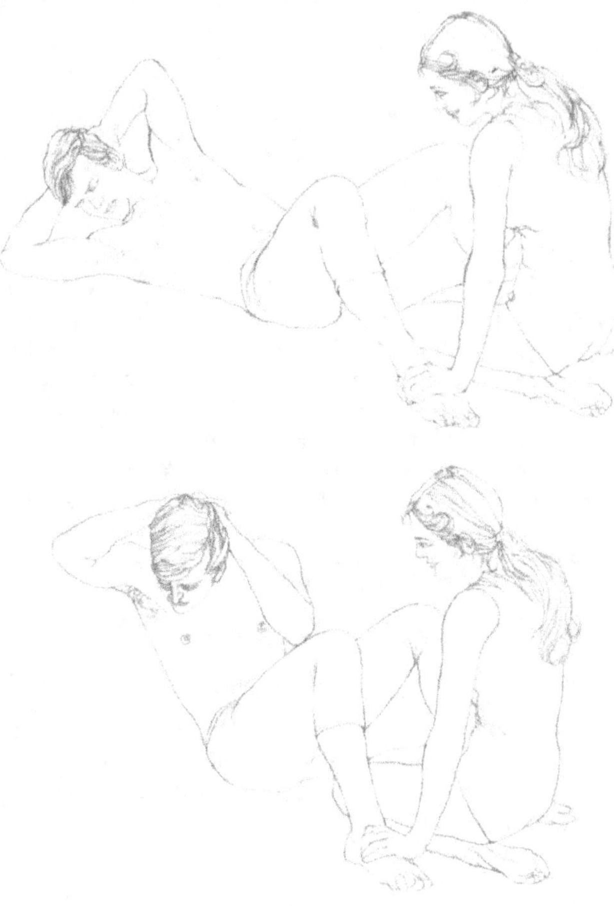

sit-up position. Your left elbow will be leading—slide it *outside* of your right knee. Maintain the twist as you roll back down to land as you started, on the right shoulder. Roll over onto the left shoulder and repeat the rotated sit-up to the left side. Be sure your leading right elbow slides *outside* of your left knee. Roll down and repeat. Start with four and work up to ten.

53. Seesaw

Hamstring and low back flexibility (do only after warm-up)

Sit opposite each other with legs widespread. If the flexibility and leg length of both partners are comparable, both rest their feet against each other's. If one is less flexible or has shorter legs, he or she rests feet against the other's calves.

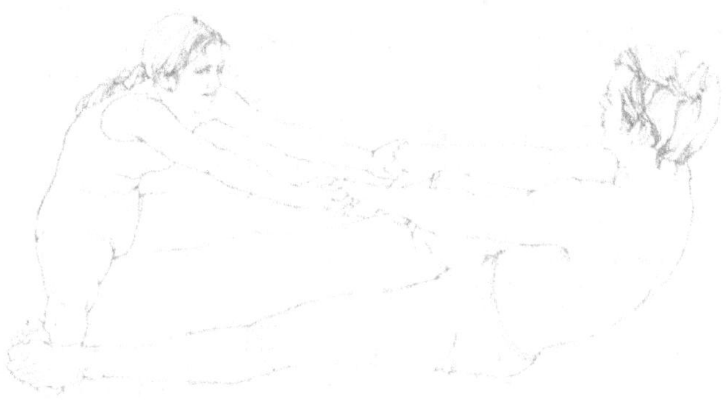

Lean forward and grasp each other's hands (this can also be done holding onto a mop handle). The pull is exerted by the one who leans backward *slowly and carefully at first.* The one being pulled concentrates and tries to let go in the tight spots. Muscles will give up tension only when they are relaxed, so be careful not to over-pull, which will cause the reverse action, tightening. Alternate for eight.

Another variation of the seesaw is the circle. One partner pulls back as before, but instead of returning to the straight-sitting position, both lean to one side, circling around as the other leans back and the first leans forward. From the lean-back–stretch-forward position, they then lean toward the other side, which circles them around again. Do four to the left and then four to the right.

54. Sit-ups to Shoulder-Touch ➤

Abdominal strengthening; hamstring stretch

One partner lies on the floor, arms overhead and feet held at the partner's waist. The standing partner leans slightly forward, placing some weight on the lying partner's feet. As the lying partner flings arms forward and reaches up, the standing partner, with legs straight, leans forward and down. The object is to have the reaching partner touch both hands to the leaning partner's shoulders and then drop back. On the second reach, the right hand crosses over to touch the partner's right shoulder. On the third, the left hand crosses over to touch the left shoulder. These three touches make up a set. Start with one and work up to four.

55. Low Back and Hamstring Stretch (only after warm-up) ➤

One partner takes the spread-leg position seated on the floor and leans straight forward, keeping knees stiff and feet slightly turned out. The other partner presses downward on the shoulders in eight easy bounces. The person who is being "stretched" tries to concentrate on the tight spots and let go. After eight bounces, sit straight for a second or two and repeat. Do four.

The exercises for stretch employing another person's help will get faster results than those in which each person must do his or her own pulling to stretch. That is because the whole body can relax while someone else is doing the work. There is another facet at work here, two in fact. One is trust. The person being "stretched" knows the other is *feeling* the reaction of the stretch through pressing hands and will know when to stop. The other is sensitivity. The pressing hands must have knowledge in them, *something* must tell them when enough is enough. This can be developed. Try for it.

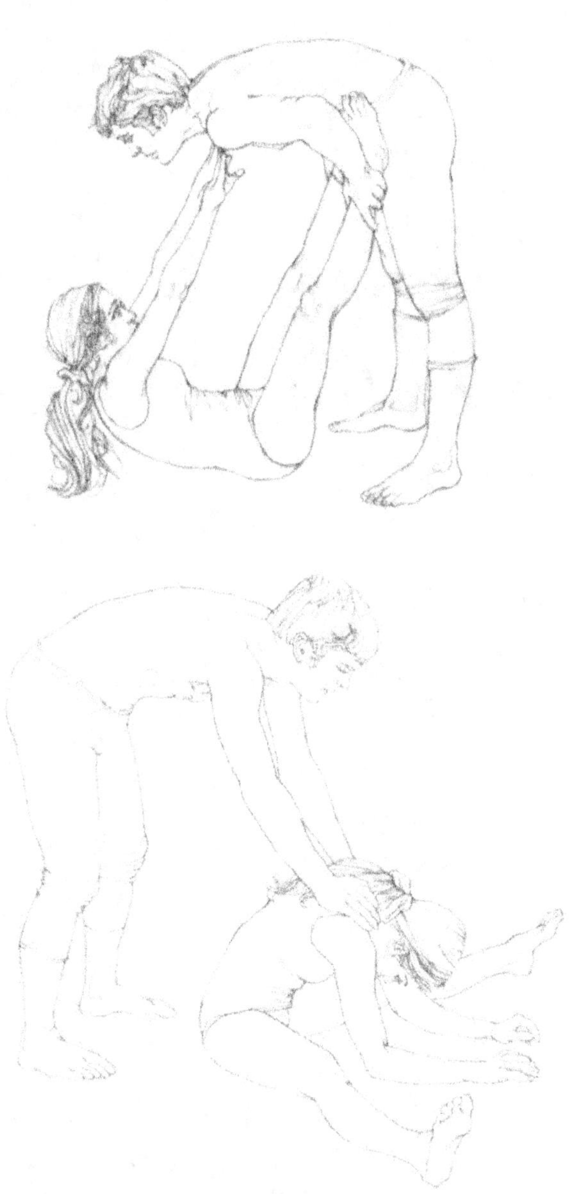

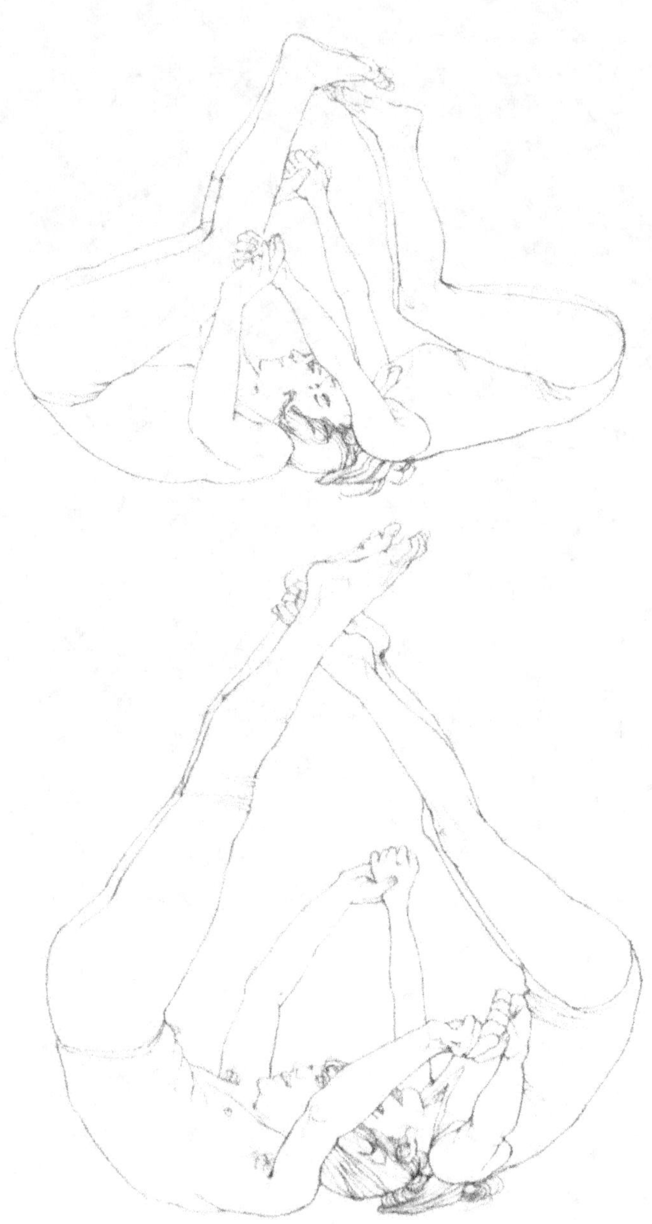

◄

56. The Pyramid

Abdominal strength

Lie supine, head to head, and grasp hands (this can also be done holding onto a mop handle). Each partner, using the support of the other, curls first to a knee-bent position in which the legs of both come together with feet touching. Maintain the foot contact as you straighten the legs to the pyramid. Curl down and unroll to stretch out, as in the starting position. Try to get higher and higher onto the shoulders, as strength and control improve.

Later, when you are able, start in the stretched-out position, curl to the knee-bent position, straighten to the pyramid, return to the curled knee bend, and then straighten to another pyramid. Work up to six.

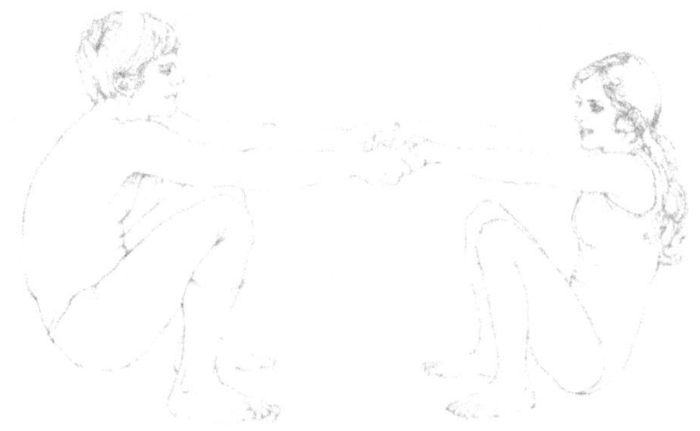

57. Flatfoot Knee Bend

Strengthens quadriceps (thigh muscles); stretches soleus (heel cord)

Stand facing each other, holding hands or holding onto a mop handle. With feet facing straight forward and legs either slightly apart or together, use each other's pull to do a full knee bend with heels on the floor. Start with four and work up to twenty, trying to depend less and less on the partner's balancing pull. This will happen only if you make an effort to stretch the heel cords.

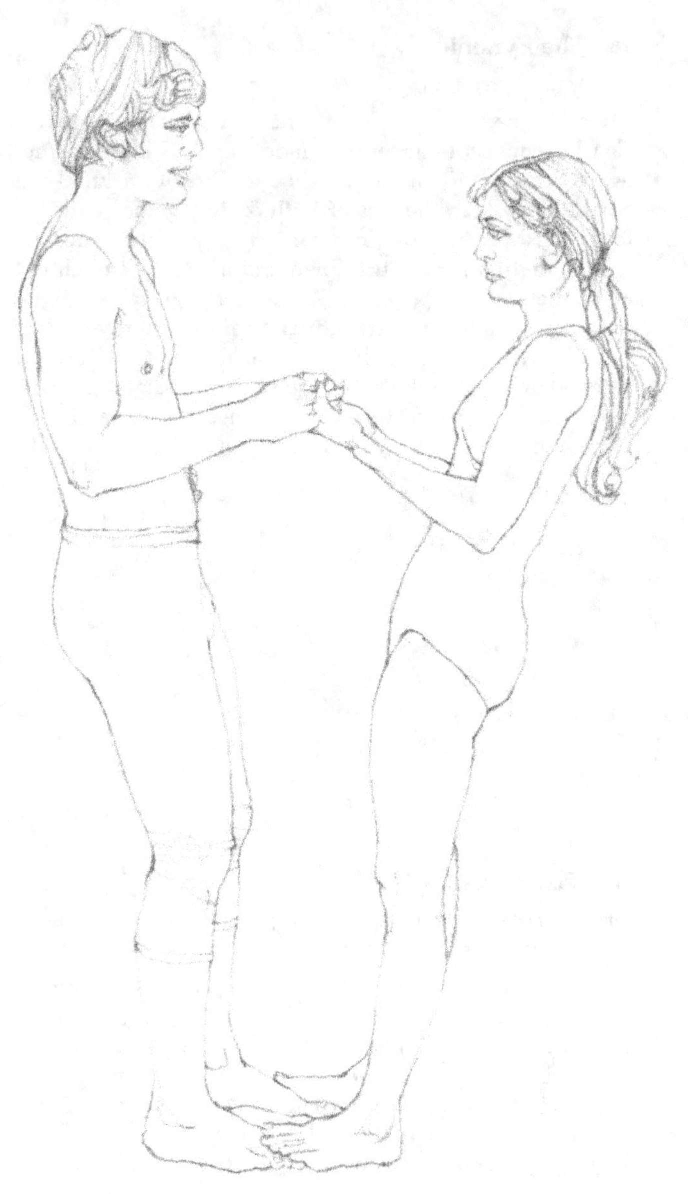

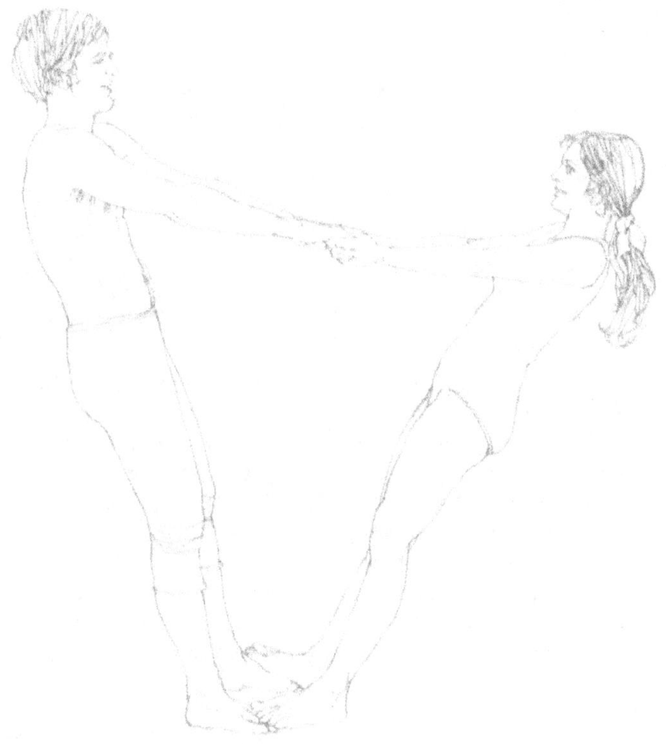

58. Pull-back Knee Bend

Quadriceps, arms, hands, shoulders, and back

Stand facing each other, holding hands. Keeping your heels flat on the floor, feet slightly apart for balance, and the toes of the lighter partner on top of the toes of the other, lean back. When arms are at full stretch, lower into

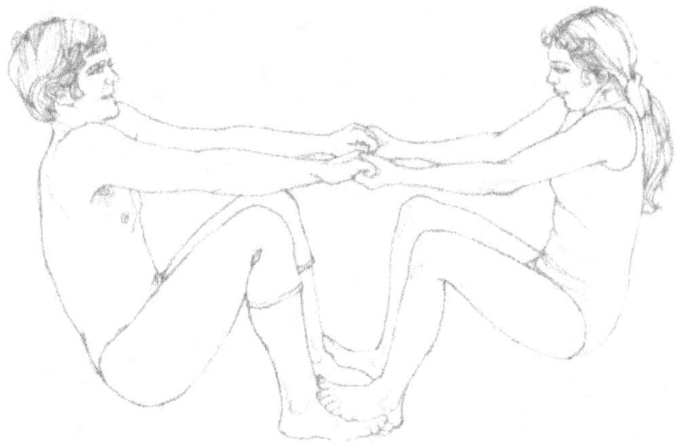

a deep knee bend. Rise again and pull in to the starting position. Start with four.

While this exercise does improve strength, its chief value lies in teaching you to *feel* and *react* to the dynamics of the other person. This is a kind of nonverbal communication in which two bodies speak to each other, giving the kind of cooperation that comes from complete awareness. Until you develop it, you certainly won't be able to hold the lean-back and descent, especially if you are of different sizes and weights.

59. Back-to-Back Knee Bend ►

Stand far enough apart to require a slight lean from both partners. Link arms and place feet slightly apart for balance. Keeping the back pressure even, go slowly down into a full knee bend and then come back up to the standing position. Do four.

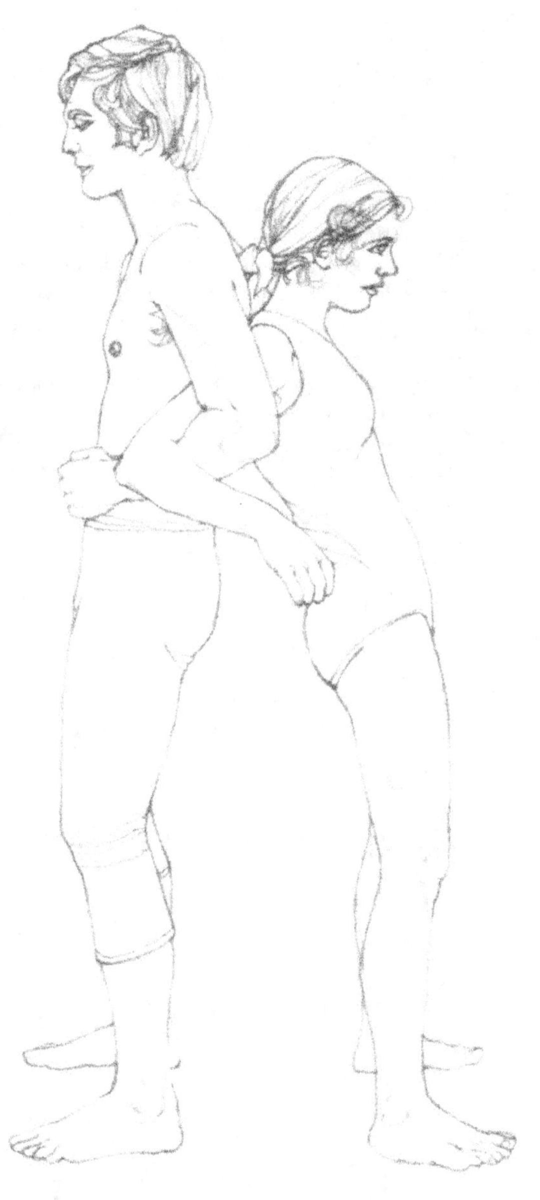

60. Pullover

Abdominal strength; back stretch; abdominal strength; balance

This is not a difficult exercise, but it does require cooperation, abdominal strength, awareness of where the body is in space, as well as awareness of your own body in relation to that of another's. It also requires the ability to give up all tension and just let the whole body hang loose. When it is done correctly, it is a cinch; when it isn't, it's grim. And the whole secret lies in bottoms.

Stand back to back, either holding hands at shoulder level or holding onto a mop handle just back of the shoulders. Now, here is the trick: the bottom of the lifter is pushed under (below) that of the partner to be

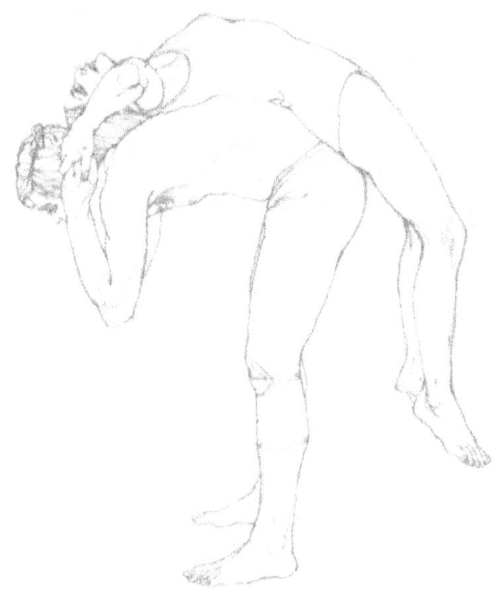

lifted. If the heights of the partners are equal, no problem. A little bend in the lifter's knees, and the proper alignment takes place. Then the lifter leans *slowly* forward until the other body hangs free and relaxed. When balance has been found, the lifter straightens his knees, and gentle stretch takes place in the back and abdominals of the body draped over his back. To set it down, the lifter merely straightens, and the other slides off.

If the girl (who is usually the weaker of the two) is smaller, it's much easier, as there need be very little knee bend, if any. She simply slides her bottom under his and leans forward. Since his weight is over ner legs, there is little strain, *as long as he doesn't fight the pull.* Try to relax and tip the head back; she probably won't drop you. Alternate one each, and work up to six.

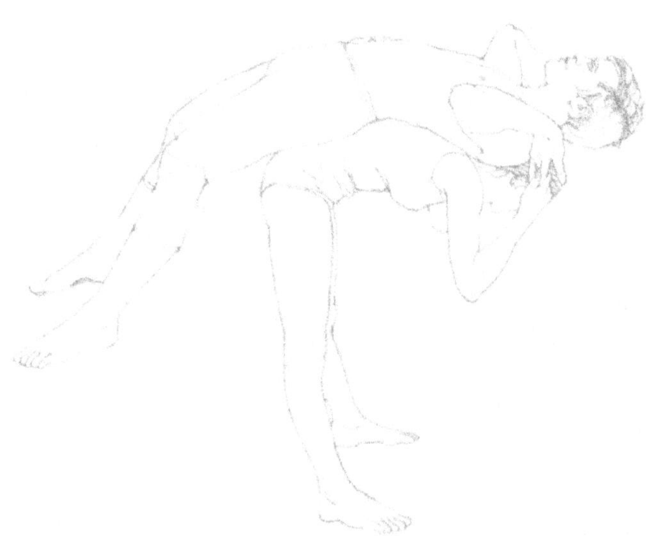

61. Push-Me, Pull-You

Strengthens arms, hands, back, abdominals, gluteals, legs, and feet; also an exercise in sensitivity

Stand with the outsides of the right feet against each other. Spread legs well for balance-and-push position. Place the right upper arms and shoulders together (don't link arms), and start to push. The weaker partner gives all she has in the push; the stronger limits his push to a holding action. Both partners will be strengthened, one to a lesser degree than the other, but the stronger partner will learn to *feel* exactly how much pressure the other can take without being either over-

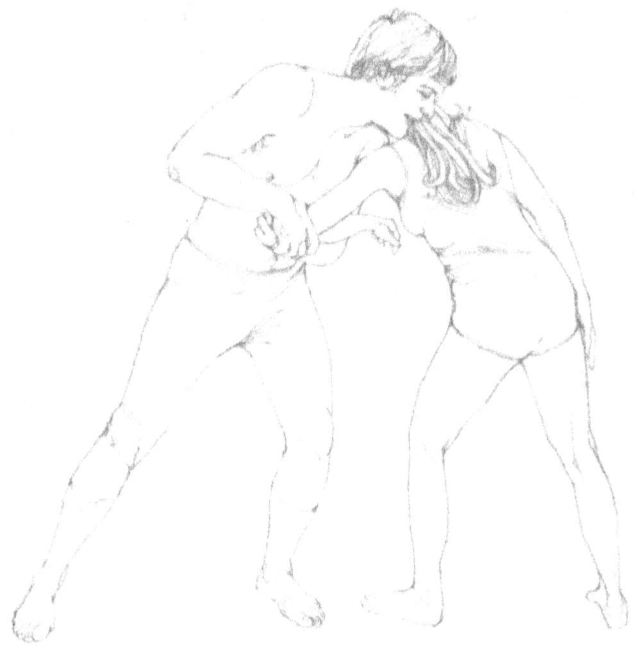

run or just plain forced to quit. Hold the push for five seconds and then reverse sides. Do one of each as one-half of a set. Go on to the next exercise to complete the set.

Keeping the outsides of the right feet pressed against each other, each partner grasps the right wrist of the other. This doubles the strength of the hold and is insurance against parting company in mid-pull. Pull against each other as hard as the strength of the weaker partner will permit. The stronger partner holds the pull steady and allows for a nicety of balance. Hold for five seconds and change sides. This makes up the second half of the set. Do four sets.

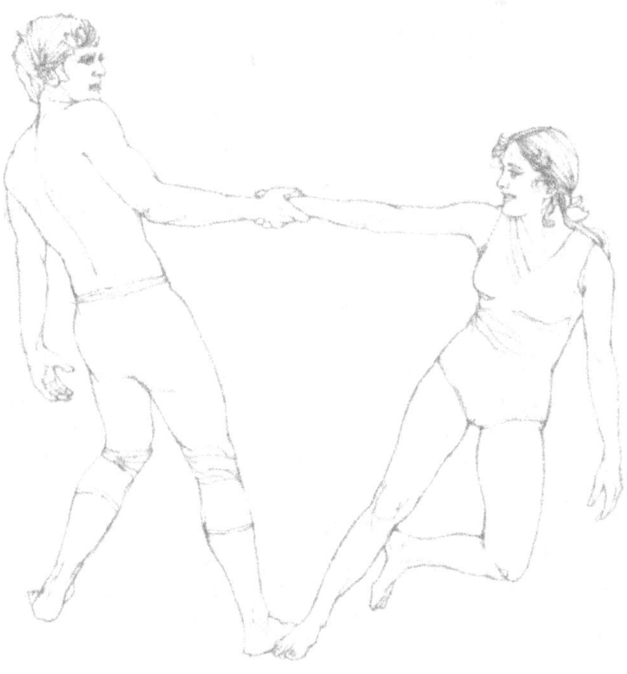

Jogging

Jogging has value. It improves the action of both heart and lungs, it strengthens legs and gluteals, and it gives feet the needed workout to release tightened muscles. Jogging can also be one of those very necessary physical outlets that release the tensions built up during the day. What's wrong with it?

Many people find jogging boring. Many people, women in particular, have never run at all, have no training in running, have no strength for running, and no interest. Many people have been discouraged from running when they started too fast, ran too far, and developed painful muscle spasms. There are neighborhoods where you simply can't run anymore, and anyway, who wants to do it alone?

There are answers to every one of those objections. Let's take the most important one first, since, if you don't correct that one, you won't run twice. *How to run.* Many people run on their toes. They never come down to rest on their heels at all, and consequently, they strain all the muscles in their feet and legs and end up in pain. That's discouraging. Check back with exercises 5 and 7 for the feet, and you will see how the weight is taken on the toes and the foot is rested when the heel again touches down. Practice those two exercises first, and then, when you start your jogging program, try to touch lightly down on the heel with each step. You will then find yourself able to bounce right back up to take off from the toe, but release will have been effected.

If you have never run, rarely run, or haven't run in a long time, your running muscles will be out of shape. No matter how much urging you get from family and friends, don't start out fast, go far, or keep it up long. You *can* if you want to, but you won't enjoy it. And if you have no experience in it, you may think that that's the way it's supposed to feel—agonizing. Not so. When you are in shape for it, you feel good while you are running, and you feel good after you have run. And you feel *wonderful* the next day. If you are going to run out-of-doors, start with walking. First, set yourself a one-mile course. Usually about eleven blocks in the city. If you live in suburbia or the country, use the speedometer in your car to mark it. If you don't have a car, measure your own stride and find out how many such strides you need to cover a mile (5,280 feet). Mark the distance at start and finish—and you are ready.

When walking the mile feels comfortable (walking that mile once a day for a month will take off or keep off one solid pound of fat—that's twelve pounds a year) *then* start your running. Run ten steps and walk fifty for the first few days. After a week, up your running steps to fifteen, twenty if you feel comfortable, but keep your walking steps at fifty. Week by week, push your running steps up until you reach the fifty-fifty level; then, start decreasing the walking steps. One day you will be running the full mile without walking, and it will be totally painless.

Running in place indoors can be just as great a disaster as taking off after the town's prize jogger for a nice evening's jaunt of ten miles. The idea of running five hundred steps in place is dangerous—for this reason. You use the same set of muscles in exactly the same way, five hundred times in quick succession. The cross-country runner, even the jogger running along the lane, uses the muscles differently and even brings in other muscles in order to accommodate the uneven terrain. The floor offers no such variety when you run in place. Therefore *you* must offer the variety. You can limit your running by counting, but that's pretty dull. A better way is to use music and sets of different types of foot and leg exercises in running patterns.

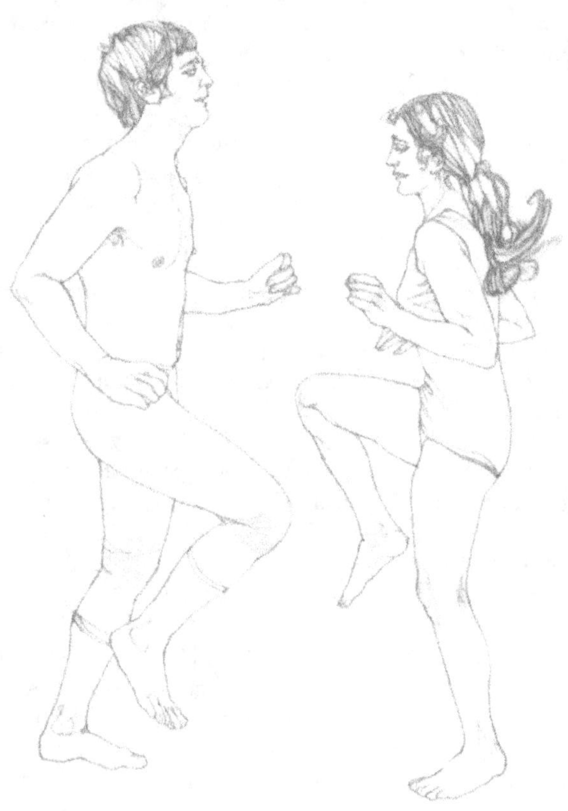

62. Running Series

Plain run. Run in place for sixteen steps, being sure to land on your toes and to touch down for a fleeting second with the heels.

High knee lift. For the next sixteen counts, lift the knees high as you try to stretch the insteps by pointing your toes. Don't forget the heel touchdown.

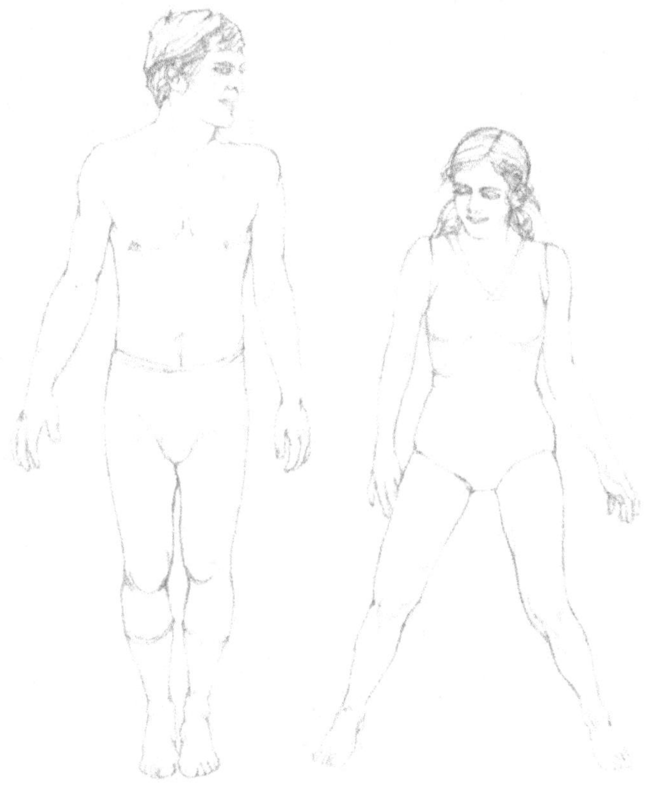

Apart-together. Jump both feet apart and together to sixteen counts. This will force the sides of the feet and legs to participate, and it will change the way your weight falls onto your running muscles.

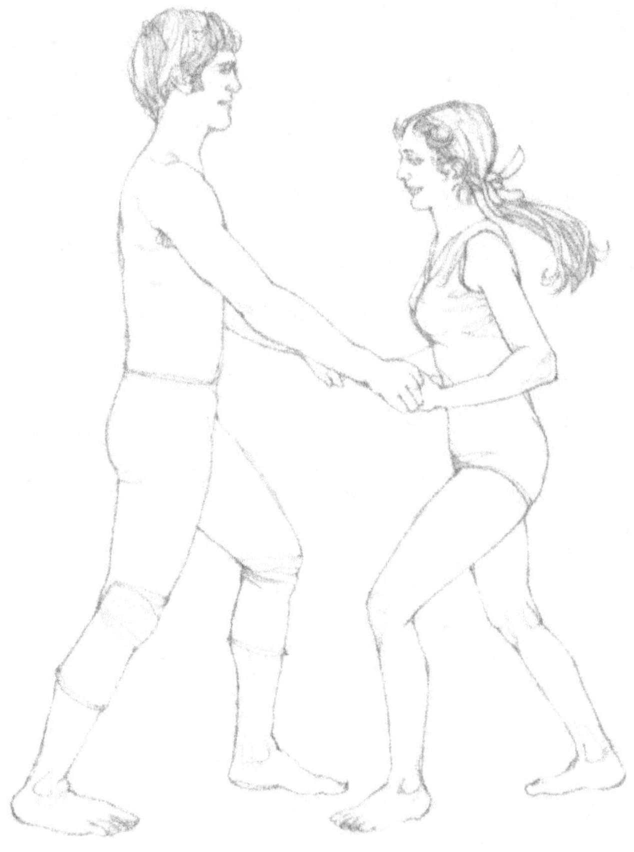

Scissors. Scissor both feet past each other for sixteen counts. This is in contrast to both the straight down-up motion and the side-to-side. Running muscles must adapt to an entirely different attack.

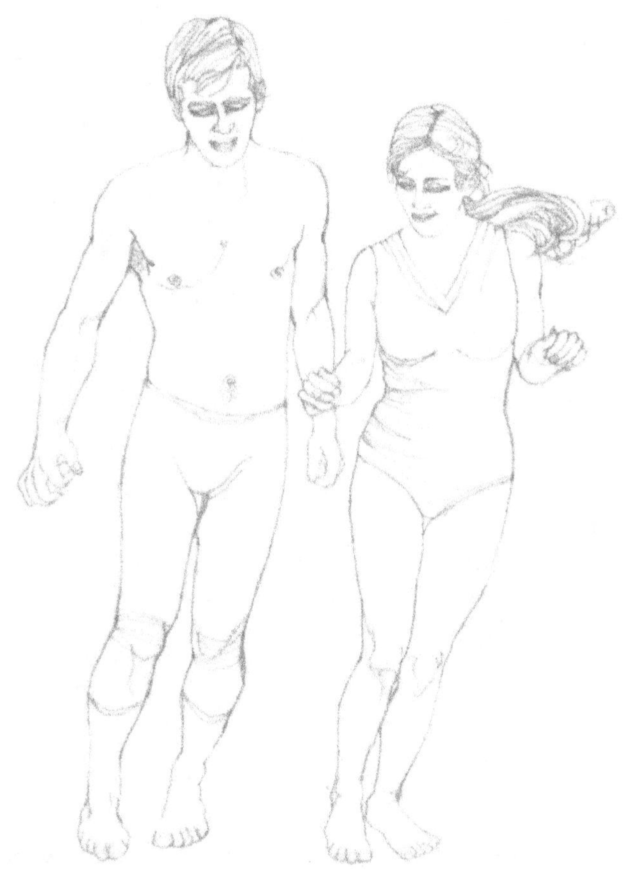

Side-to-side. Jump both feet from side to side for a count of sixteen.

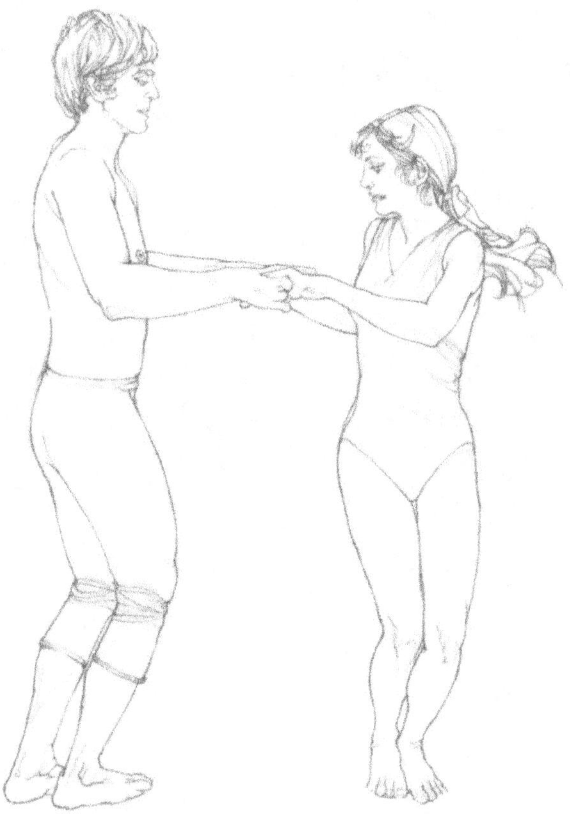

Twist. Twist the body left and right from the waist down. Be sure to keep the chest facing straight forward, or even twist a little in opposition to the feet. Count to sixteen.

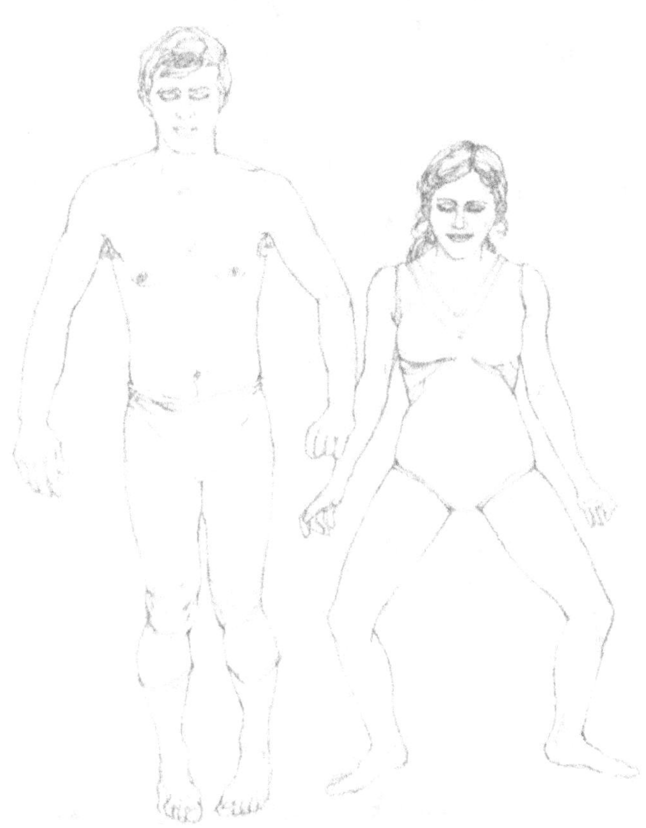

In-and-out. Jump the feet so that the toes come close to meeting as the feet turn in. Then jump the legs wide as you turn the feet outward. Do sixteen.

Forward and back kick-ups. Finish up with eight kick-ups in front and eight kick-ups to the back, for one set. Do four sets.

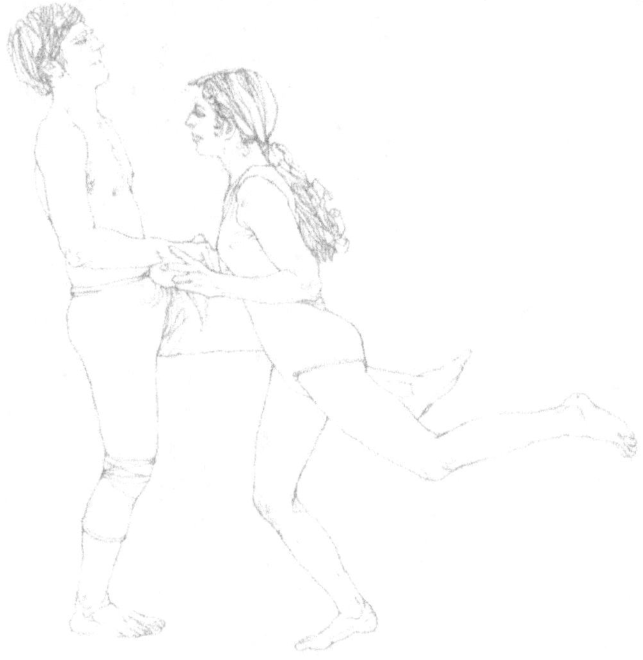

If you are a rank beginner, you'll never make it through all of that. So put on a record with a good fast beat, and do just one movement. In a day or so, add a second and still later a third, until you finally have them all. That still won't take a whole pop record. So when you come to the end of your series, if the record is still going, start over.

Strength

There are two ways to increase strength and at least a hundred reasons for doing so. The reasons for doing so run the entire gamut from being better at your favorite sport, improving your appearance, getting through childbirth quickly and easily . . . to having more fun longer and oftener in bed. Take your pick, and get started.

The two ways you can improve strength are by repetition of a given *correct* movement and by movement against resistance. If your tennis serve is a good one and you practice it over and over, it will improve. If your serve is of the backyard variety and does not utilize your full potential, you can repeat it hours daily for months and you will always merely pop the ball over. Even if the movement is correctly done—say, the bent-knee sit-up, with feet held down—repetition has its drawbacks. It's both boring and damaging to skin if you have to do two hundred to get a good abdominal-muscle workout. One of the best answers to that problem is resistance.

Exercise 61 is an example of resistance, using the strength of two people working against each other's strength. Swimming is an example of resistance found in working against water. You can do the running series in water and have the benefit of plenty of resistance. You can also use weight bags.

Weight bags are the easy, sensible way to create resistance, because they can be used in so many different ways, but if you already own barbells, don't give them to the Salvation Army. They can be used in exactly the same way as the weight bags in the following series.

To make weight bags, use either sand or lead shot. While shot costs more, it is far easier to handle, store, and make into bags. In order to differentiate the weights easily, use colored denim, which both wears well and is very attractive. Yellow denim rectangles measuring 6½ inches by 11 inches will do nicely for one-pounders. Red denim in 10-by-12-inch rectangles will hold two pounds, and blue denim rectangles of 10 inches by 13 inches will hold five pounds. You will need two of each for a basic set.

WEIGHT BAG
Use pins to hold shot while stitching.

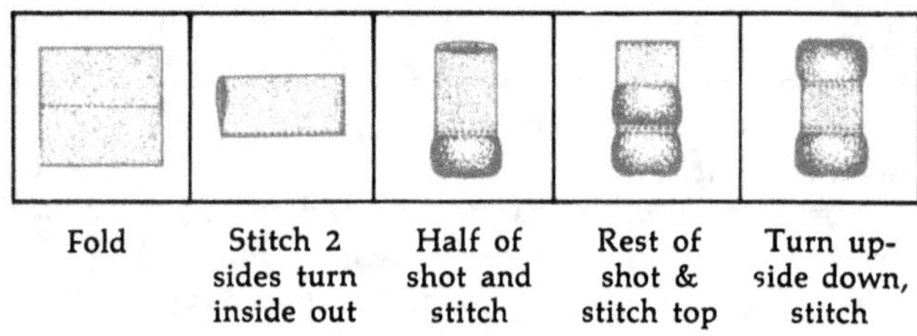

Use a mop handle, broomstick, or dowel on which to drape as many weight bags as you can handle *easily*. If you are a starter and have barbells handy, take all the weights off and use only the bar. It usually weighs about twenty pounds (a little heavier than your improvised set).

63. Clean to Chest and Press ►

Exercises 63–65 make up a set.

(*a*) Lean forward and pick up your weights. (*b*) As you stand erect, bring the weights to your chest and then press them overhead. Return them to your chest and then lower them until they are hanging in front of your thighs, and your arms are at full stretch.

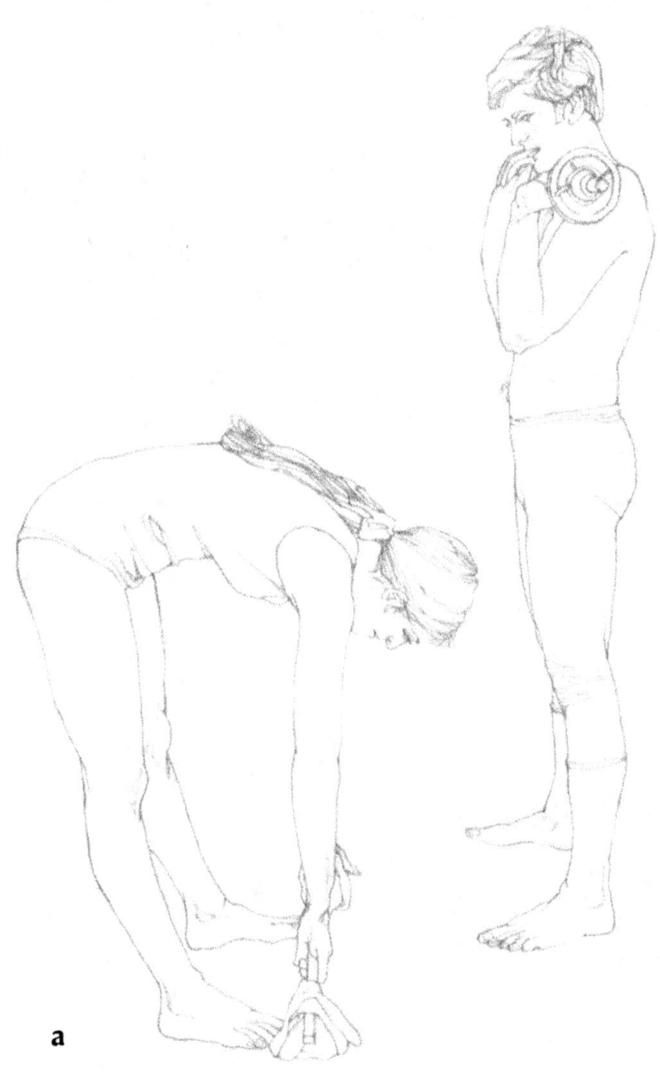

a

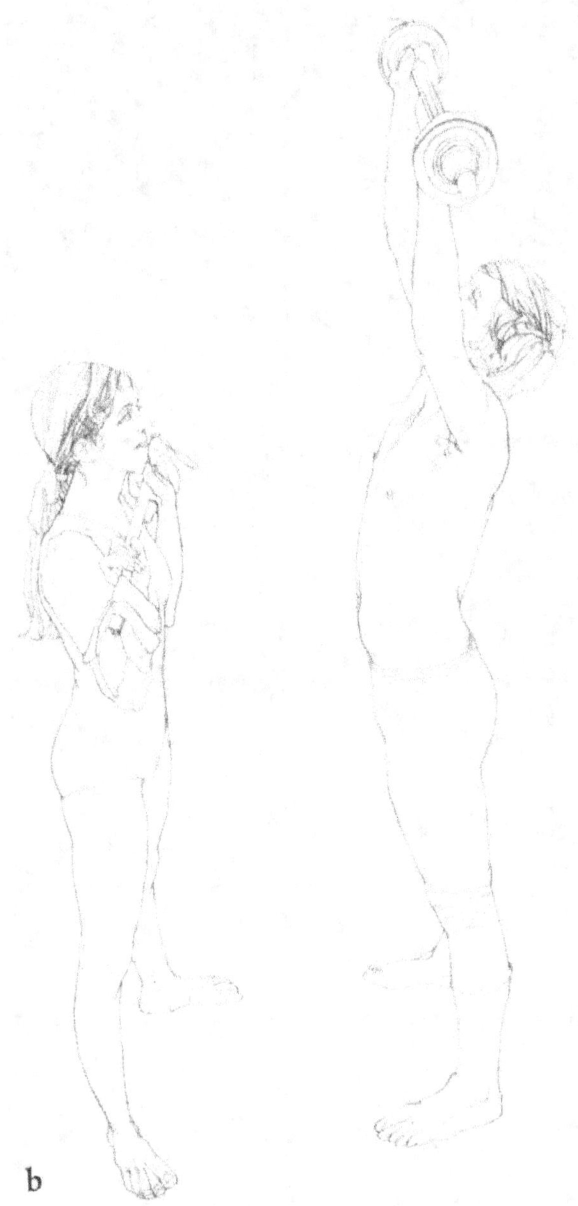
b

64. Reverse Curl

Bring the weights to your chest again and lower to the thigh hang. Keep your elbows in and down. Do two, and then set your weights on the floor and reverse your hands. Stand up with the weights in the thigh-hang position. This is the second exercise in the set.

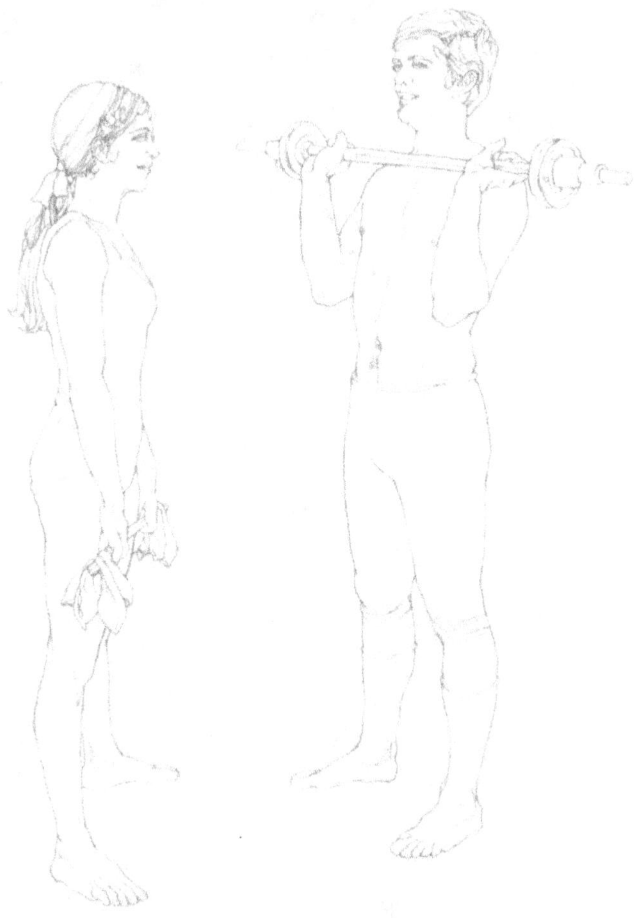

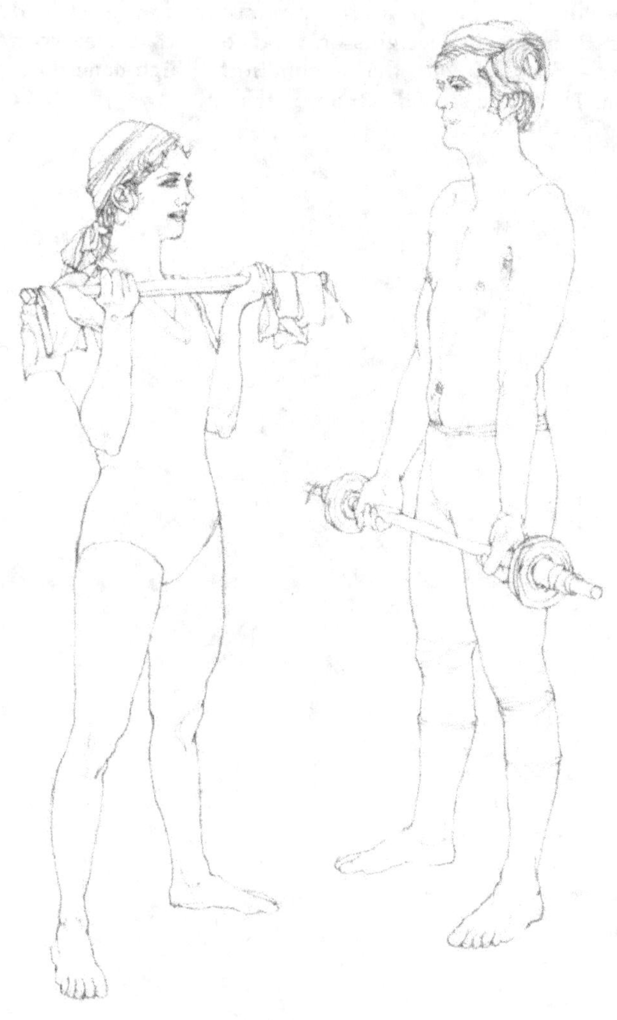

◄

65. Curl

Curl your arms inward to bring the weights to your chest, then lower to the thigh hang. Do two. Replace the weights on the floor and reverse your hands.

Do three of these three-exercise sets.

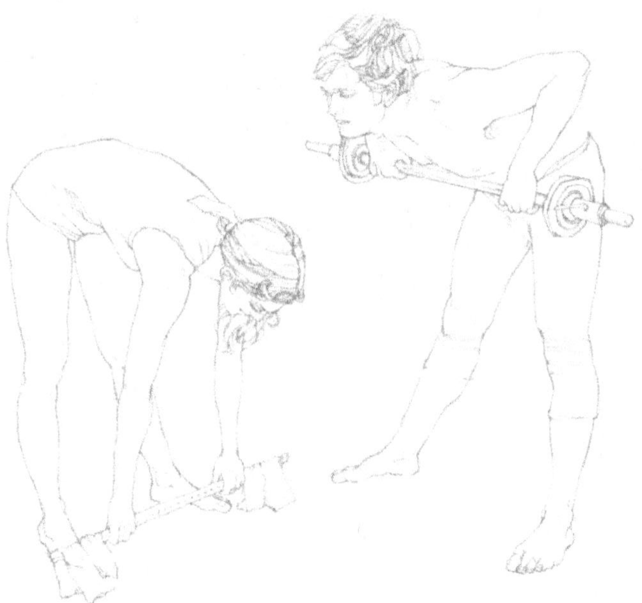

66. Bent-Over Row

With feet well apart and knees straight, lean forward from the hips and lift the weights just clear of the floor. Then, keeping your back level, bring the weights to the chest and lower to full arm stretch ten times.

67. Supine Press

Lie supine and hold weights close to your shoulders. Press them up toward the ceiling, and after your arms are at full stretch, push a little harder so that the backs of your shoulders clear the floor. Lower and repeat ten times.

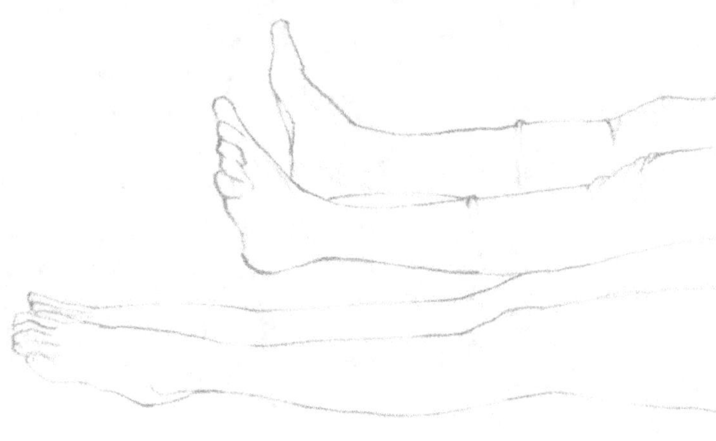

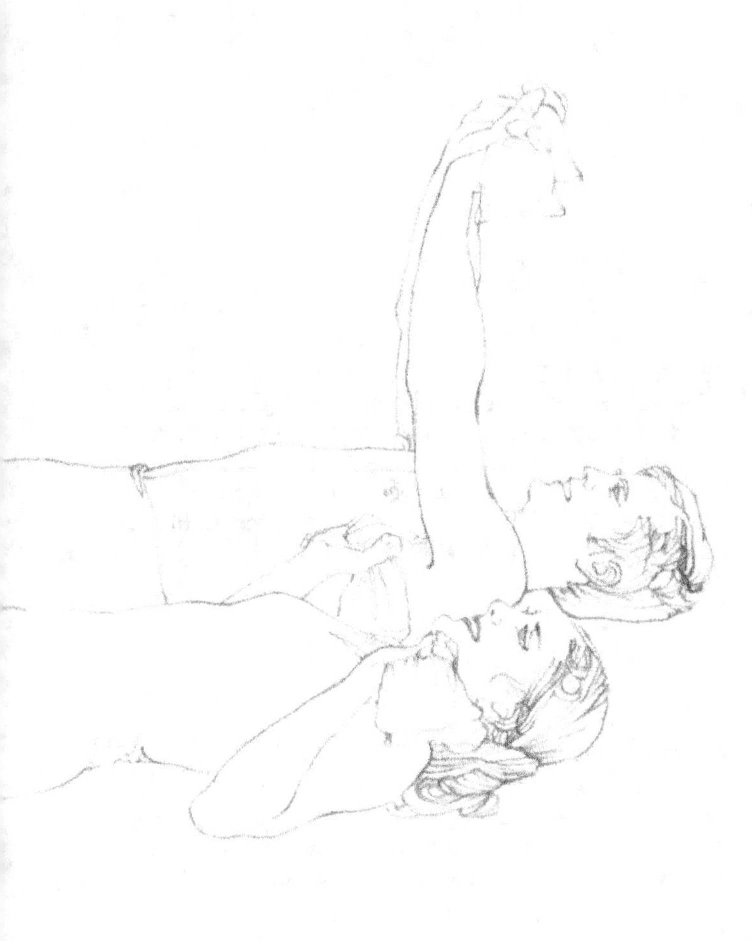

68. Pullover ➤

Lie supine and raise your weights straight above your face to full arm stretch. Lower the weights with straight arms until they *almost* touch the floor above your head. Then raise them again to the starting position above your face. Lower them with straight arms until they *almost* touch your thighs. Do ten.

69. Lateral Lift ➤

(Remove weights from dowel.) Lie supine, with weights again held with straight arms above your face. Lower both arms to the sides until the weights *almost* touch the floor. Carry them up to the starting position again. Do ten.

70. Weighted Bend and Extend ➤

Rest back on your elbows with weights hanging from your ankles. Bring one bent knee to your nose and then extend the leg straight forward, about two inches above the floor. Do eight with that leg, and then the same exercise with the other leg. Repeat three times.

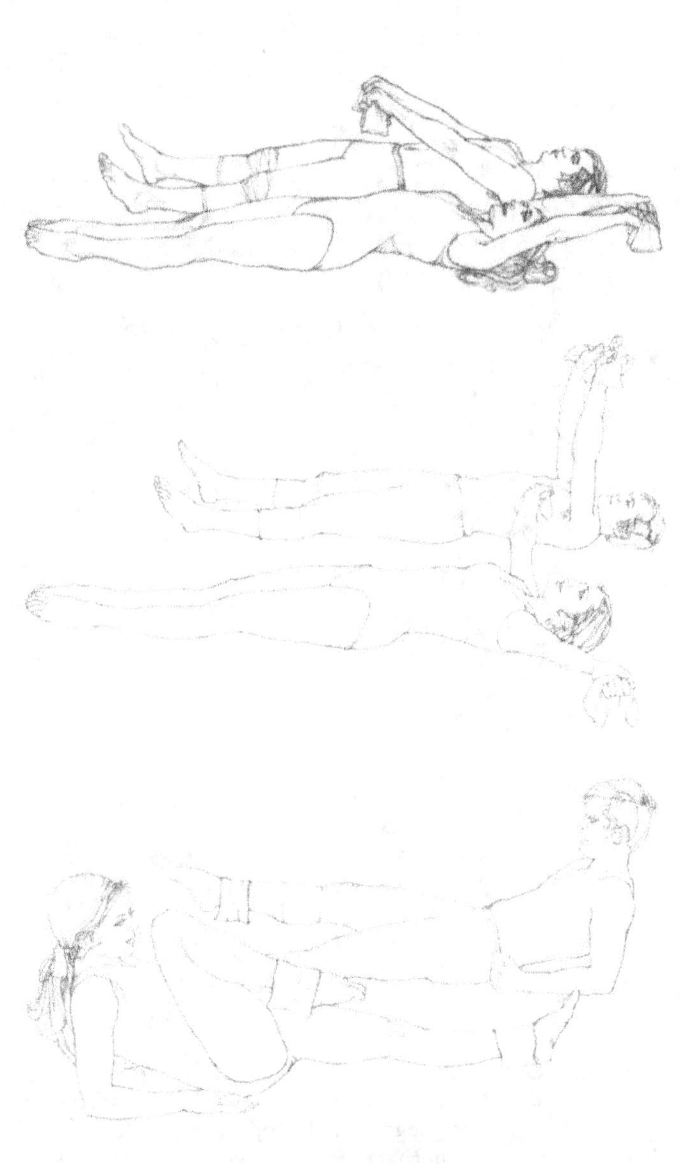

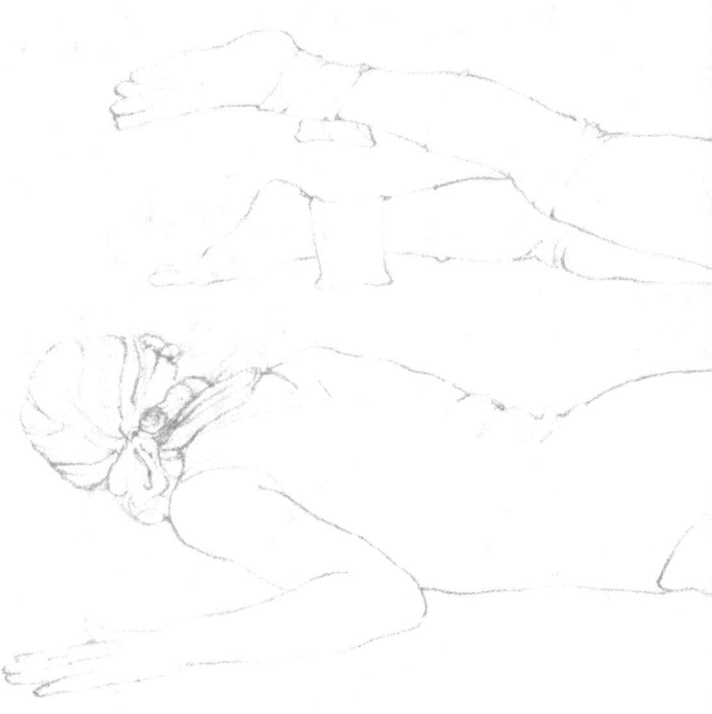

71. Prone Leg Lifts

Lie prone with weights draped over your ankles. First, with legs close together, lift one straight leg and then the other. Alternate for sixteen counts. Next,

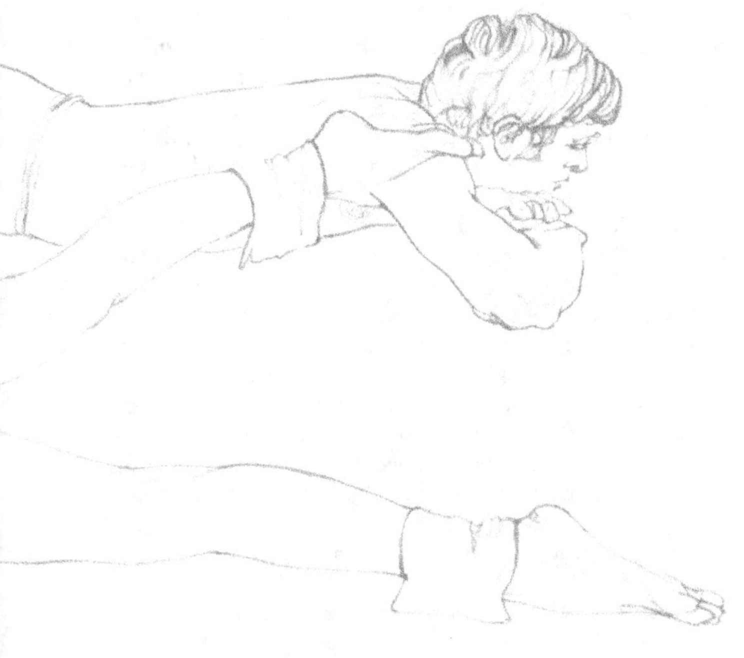

spread both legs wide, and maintaining the spread, lift first one leg and then the other. Alternate for sixteen counts.

72. Cables

Any program begs for variety, and there are many simple ways of providing it without spending a lot of money for expensive equipment. A very good way to develop strength, flexibility, and sensitivity is with the use of 1½-inch-wide strips of nylon or cotton webbing, found in curtain and drapery shops. Two strips six feet in length will provide an excellent piece of equipment. Sew the ends back on themselves to make wrist holds. You should be able to slip your hands through easily. One partner thrusts hands through the two ends of his cable, and then the other partner threads her cable through the circle made by the cable and her partner's hands. She then slips her own hands through her cable ends. This makes two closed links of a chain. You could use ropes, but holding onto rope ends would tire hands very quickly, long before the arms would tire. Wrist cuffs allow the arms, back, adominal, and legs to be pushed much farther.

(*a*) Start by facing each other with legs well spread and hands resting on thighs. The cables between the two partners should be barely taut. Raise the arms from the thighs and carry them sideward as you lean backward, each supporting the other's weight. This will mean much more lean for the lighter partner; and therefore greater sensitivity to his partner must be experienced by the supporting partner if the balance is to be maintained. This balance can be maintained by spreading the arms wider or narrowing the spread. Only practice will teach you how.

(*b*) Then bring the hands in toward each other as you lean still farther back.

(*c*) Cross one arm over the other as you bend forward from the hips. Be sure to keep the pull constant and the arms straight. When your back is parallel with the floor, keep your head down and raise both arms wide. The pull in your shoulders will be considerable, so begin gently and be aware of the other person's flexibility or lack of it. *Don't overpull.*

Return to the starting position, going back the same way you came, bringing arms downward and inward in a circle across your body. And as you stand straight, open wide and lean back.

This is only a sample of how cables can be used. You will find many others, from deep knee bends to forward leans while facing out. The cables stretch both upper back and chest muscles and strengthen every muscle brought into play to support the lean. Use slow music and make every effort to increase resistance by leaning farther and harder as skill improves.

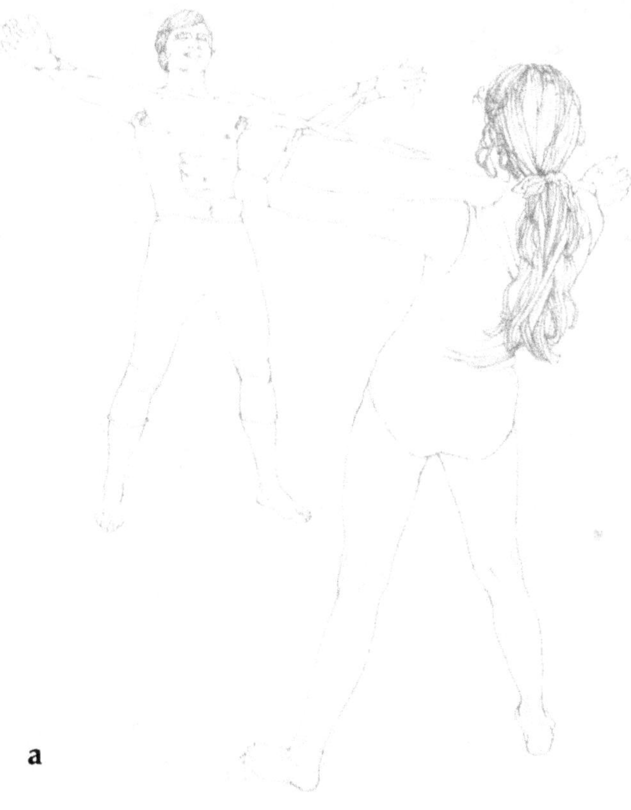

a

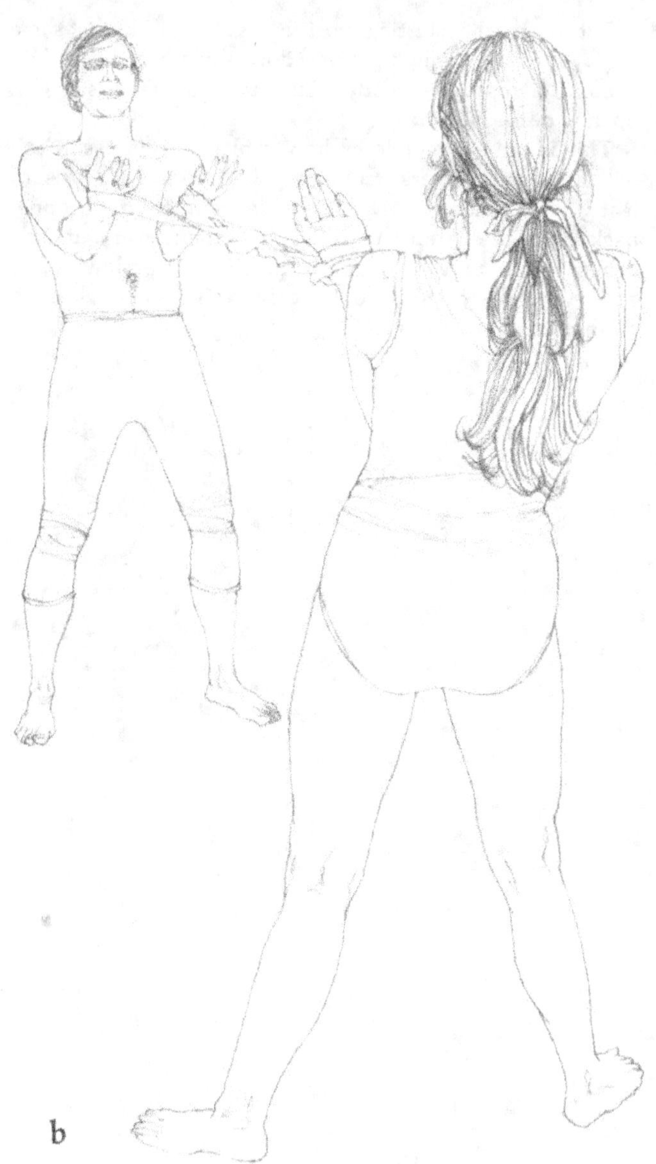

b

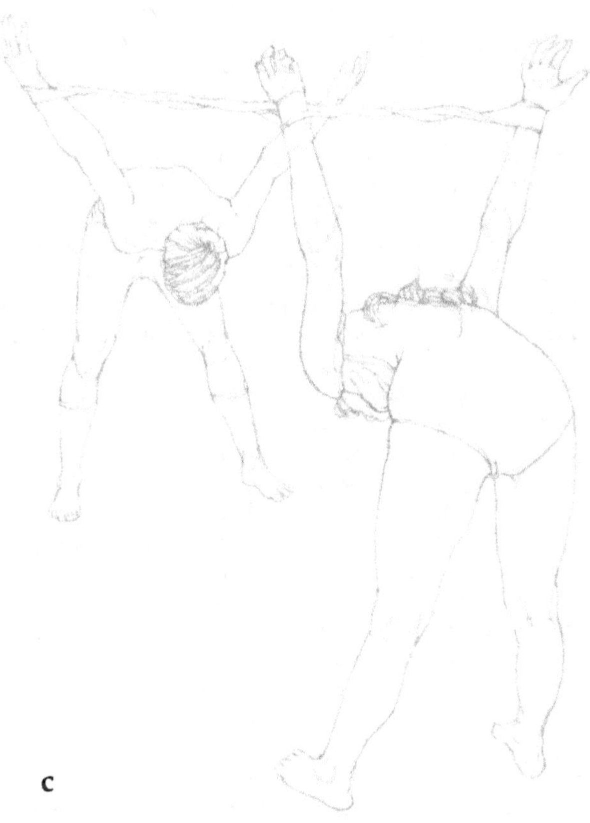

c

Meditation and Relaxation

In recent years Eastern philosophies have been embraced by Western peoples to a degree no one would have believed possible a generation ago. Yoga and other disciplines are as common as classes in public speaking in schools. Even in YMCAs and YWCAs, as well as in other centers, meditation is so commonplace that one no longer wonders if the man who seems to be sleeping while sitting up in the train may miss his stop. He's probably meditating and knows exactly when the train will reach his hometown. Boys taking lessons in karate also practice meditation, high-school girls join meditation groups as part of their psychology classes, thousands meditate in growth centers. Why?

For some, it is to get their heads together after unpleasant side trips into the drug scene. For others, it is a search for some kind of peace in a world grown too complicated. For many it is blessed relaxation of mind and body. There are as many reasons as there are meditators, but the one that concerns us here is the effect of meditation on relaxation. Without question, it is a distinct aid. If you want to test this theory, try this experiment. Practice several of the exercises previously described, enough to be called a good workout. Then, after doing the following relaxation-meditation combination, again do the same exercises, and notice what a genuine contribution this makes in bringing release to a tense, tired body. The benefits of such release are similar in kind, though not in degree, to those provided by true meditation. This exercise is but a preliminary step in easing your body and mind into a state conducive to meditation, and leading you into its elementary stages; but whether you plan to take up meditation seriously or not, the rewards of this exercise are immediate and obvious.

Sit cross-legged on the floor, with relaxed arms resting on your knees. Tip your head back and close your eyes. Breathe in deeply, and then slowly release your breath. As you release it, try to feel heavy and slow in your movements. While your breath leaves your body, bend slowly forward and let the bend in your chest force the last vestige of air from your lungs. When they are empty, hang there with head down, trying to find any tight places in back or neck. See if you can count to ten before you feel the need to breathe again. As you breathe in, slowly straighten your back, open your rib cage wide to permit a really huge volume of air to enter, and tip your head back. Repeat this deep breathing, almost totally expelling all air three times when you begin (more would make you dizzy). Then lie prone with head resting on your arms. (If you have a problem back, you will find that bending a knee out to the side takes the strain away.)

Repeat the breathing exercises in the prone position. You will have to work harder to fill your lungs, which means you will be working against resistance—always helpful—but your exhalation will be aided by the weight

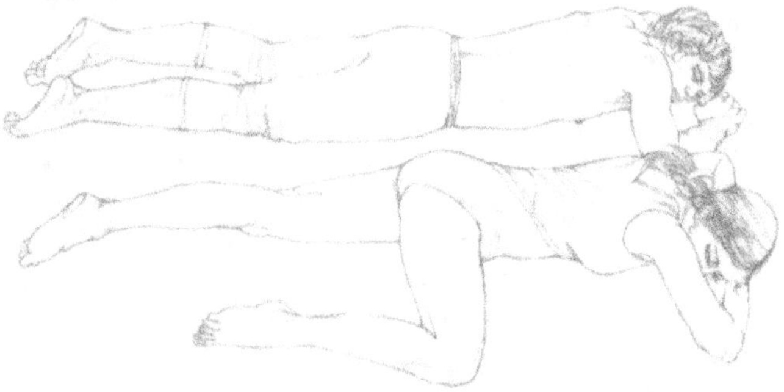

of your body on your rib cage. Since very few people ever completely empty the used air from their lungs, this too is helpful. Start with three deep breaths. Then roll onto your side.

In the side-lying position, continue with your deep breathing, but since you are lying on one side, the ribs on that side will not be able to open as wide as those on the top side. One side will take in more air than the other. Pay attention to it and try to force even more air into that side. Do three, and then roll to the other side. Repeat the breathing once more, and then roll onto your back.

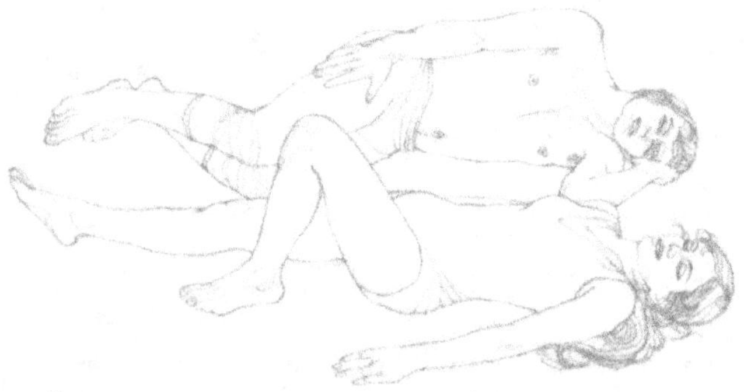

If you have a problem back, lying supine may be a strain. Raise one knee if you must, but only if you must. Fold your arms across your chest and take in one more huge breath; then, allowing the air to escape through your teeth in a hiss, squeeze all the air from your lungs. Take two more quiet breaths with arms relaxed at your sides and begin the following litany:

Relax your head
The back of your neck is resting
Your shoulders are resting
Let go in your upper arms
Your elbows

Relax your lower arms
Wrists
Hands
Fingers

Inhale quietly . . . and exhale
Inhale . . . exhale

Your back is resting
Let go in your waist
Relax your hips
The backs of your thighs
Knees
Calves
Ankles
Insteps
Feet
Toes
Inhale quietly . . . exhale
Inhale . . . exhale

Now, before you repeat those words, become aware of the top of your head and then the soles of your feet. All of you, everything that has to do with you, lies between those two points. Find them and *know* where they are. Notice the feel of the floor against whatever parts of you touch it. Try to feel as though those parts become one with the floor. Notice where your knees are and where your legs join your body. If there is any tightness in your back, let go. Find your hands and "think warmth" into them (it is entirely possible to do so). Now, notice your ears and try accurately to measure, not in inches but in space, the distance between them. Then notice your closed eyes. Focus on them and become aware of where they are, and then, with eyes still closed, try to look into another room just in front of you. Then relax and start the litany again. If you have time, don't get up immediately. Just lie there and float. When you feel you must get up, tell yourself that you are completely relaxed and that you are going to stay that way. Then raise your hands above your head to rest on the floor and start to stretch. Think how the cat stretches. Grow longer and longer. Stretch your legs and point your toes; grow and grow. When you reach full stretch, hold it for a couple of seconds—and then let go!

When you first start this, take turns—one doing the relaxing, and the other reading all the instructions right through to the end. After a few such "lessons," you will be able to do it silently by yourself.

Relaxation can be sought at any time, but you will soon find that if you exercise first, your level of rest will be deeper and the degree of relaxation much greater. Your mind knows that your body needs surcease from tension, so enlist the help of that body in aiding itself, through physical outlets. There will come a time when that body is so patterned to relax in this manner that all you will have to do after exercise is lie down—and it will all happen automatically.

7

Self-Image

You tell a great deal about *the way you think and feel about yourself* by the way you sit, stand, walk, run, shake hands, hold your head, move your eyes, place your arms. But you may not be entirely correct in your interpretation of yourself and may, in fact, be quite different from the person you portray.

Where does the self-image come from? It comes from feedback from other people, and this feedback draws its strength from our relationship to those other people. I can well remember my mother saying she was so glad my sister had my father's nose. She thought hers was "terrible." So often she would tell us how her favorite teacher was overheard to say, "My! That Nell would be a beautiful girl if it weren't for her terrible nose." Well, to begin with, her nose wasn't "terrible." It was snubbed and it suited her face, and she was very lovely in a way she never suspected. She wanted to be "elegant" and she was actually piquant, but no one ever told her which way her looks really went. She only knew that she missed being elegant, and she blamed it on her nose.

The most important person where feedback is concerned is mother. Feedback begins when we do, and the feedback is present even before first meeting on this side of the womb. Even the tiniest baby knows if it is well loved and welcome. It also knows when it is neither, which may explain some inexplicable behavior in children.

When we are little children, we may not understand

the words grown-ups use in reference to our behavior, appearance, and personalities, but we rarely miss their import. The younger we are, the fewer criteria we have with which to judge, and so we accept them. Sometimes we spend a whole lifetime trying to prove them to be right—and we don't even know we are doing it. Let me show you how it works.

Like most children, I had two parents who provided the feedback that would at least start my self-evaluation. I also had a very beautiful little sister who was a "good girl." Comparisons are indeed odious, for they are sure to cause a certain amount of discomfort to one of the parties. When they are made often enough, that discomfort becomes chronic. In order to make the discomfort bearable, the condition has somehow to be reversed, if only in the mind of the sufferer.

I was about four when I realized that grown-ups were always exclaiming over my sister's beauty, which was indeed truly unusual. After going on at length about her they would suddenly remember me and, turning smiles toward me, they would exclaim "And this one's so *healthy*!" I hadn't the slightest idea what *healthy* meant, but I knew all about pretty, beautiful, lovely, charming, and adorable. None of those adjectives were ever applied to me, so I supposed at that early age that I wasn't any of those things. I held on to that so tenaciously that it took until my thirty-fifth birthday (to the day) to part me from it. I didn't have to rely on a "terrible nose" to reinforce my feelings about myself, not I. I had something far more reliable—my character. I was just plain bad. It was true, in a way. I was into everything. I took things apart, I entered houses closed for the season, I "borrowed" things like tools and paint, grapes from a neighbor's arbor, apples from a convent garden, other kids' bikes. And periodically, I ran away. Roughly three times a day I was asked why I couldn't be "good" like my sister. Well, what's not good? Bad. So I sure worked at it. What isn't beautiful? Ugly, and I worked at that too, in the clothes I wore when I chose them, and *to* the clothes I wore when someone with my fragile sister in mind chose them. What isn't "a little lady"? A roughneck, and I worked hard at that. By the time I was fourteen, in spite of ten years' training in dance, I walked across the room like a fighter coming out of his corner. It was finally decided that I would be sent to a convent, where, presumably, the rough edges would be rounded off.

The place for me would have been the not-yet-born Outward Bound School, but I had other lessons to learn. The safest way to act in a boarding school is harmless, and I didn't. While I had been growing up under the burden of my "bad" character, I had found a perfect escape, books. If I was reading, I wasn't being "bad," so I was encouraged to read as much as possible, and I did. Can you imagine the dust that was raised when I took issue with the nun in charge of English who said that Boccaccio was a man who used his gifts badly (there was that word again) by writing such things as the *Decameron?* I can still hear myself (I'd only been there a week and didn't yet know that what I was doing was very upsetting). "Oh, no, madame, the *Decameron* is a beautiful book; I read it last summer." I'd also read the life of Martin Luther "last summer," and that got me into trouble in religion. *Catherine the Great* (summer before) dropped my history mark, and then, I finally caught on. But it was too late. My classmates knew I was a maverick, and they weren't at all sure I belonged. They found many ways to let me know, and I soon got the full treatment. They played a game called "Pass the Book." One kid was the "whisperer" and she would give a book to a girl as she whispered, "Give this book to the girl with the worst figure." Silently, the book was handed to the selected girl, who didn't know why she had been so favored. But she got a chance to get back, should the reason have been critical. She handed the book to someone else who had the worst hair, was the most conceited, told the biggest lies, had the funniest walk, the heaviest legs, the biggest bottom

. . . and so on *ad infinitum.* Later, just before the bell rang for evening study hall, everyone reported why they had given the book to whom. Without question I was much in their minds, if not their hearts. *Nobody* got the book as often as I did, ever. I spent many unhappy sessions in our evening study halls wishing I could look in a mirror and see if it was all true. Two years later, when I left that school, I couldn't walk across the center of the Grand Central train station in New York but had to slink furtively around the walls, hoping no one would notice my terrible figure, ugly legs, miserable hair, and funny clothes.

Those girls were important to me. I wanted desperately to belong somewhere. My early feedback had turned me into a "bad" kid. Today I would have been considered "interesting." At the convent I was considered an "outlander," so I became one. Even my teachers weren't very helpful. "Why don't you stay with your own classmates?" got the response, "They don't want me to," which elicited the retort, "Then there must be something wrong with you." There was, but I was much older before I found out. I was in the wrong school. Two years later, after total acceptance by my classmates at Horace Mann School, and then finding a happy place in the Weidman-Humphrey dance group, I was almost healed. But I was still tender in many spots, and so shy that I wouldn't go to a party under *any* circumstances. I had begun to know my worth, but I was still so shaky that the image I projected was all mixed up.

One evening, my sister was giving a party for some of her Art Students' League friends, and I returned from rehearsal while it was still in full swing. One of the boys, the only one I knew, met me in the hall. Putting his arm around my shoulders, he drew me into the center of the living room, shouting, "Hey, everybody, come meet Jeanne's little sister. (I was two years older and three inches shorter.) "We just got shoes on her last week!" I died right there. Now, of course I know that it was intended as good-natured banter, but I have learned that only secure people can take that kind of banter in stride. The insecure find darts even where none are intended.

Nor did things improve. I married a teaser. Some teasers say things they really mean but don't want to get caught saying. They are usually so busy hiding hurts of their own that they are rarely aware of the wounds they inflict. The trouble is, if they are important to you, you believe them and begin at once living up to the image *they* lay on you. This goes on year after year. Images are laid down layer on layer over the person you *really* are, until you forget who you are, if you ever really knew.

If you aren't lucky, you go all through life thinking that you just missed being beautiful because of your "terrible nose," even though in reality you are more than just beautiful, much more. But if you are lucky, someone comes along who earns your respect and trust and he tells you some truths about yourself. They ring so clear, because they *are* true, that a rip appears in the shroud and you step forth as you really are. That's what love can do. That's what love is supposed to do.

Someone can really mirror you as you are to yourself, but you can do the same wonderful things for others, stripping away their distorted self-images and revealing the wonder that they are. As usual, prevention is better than cure, and prevention begins in the beginning. Where babies are concerned, don't even think critical thoughts near them. And with children, chide them for their misbehavior but never for their appearance, their personality, or their character. If you do, they may try all their lives to prove you are right.

Now, for *your* self-image. Is it positive or is it negative? What do you think about yourself right now? Can you remember what you thought about yourself when you were six, or sixteen? What did people say about you? What did they nickname you? How did you feel about your looks? Obviously you were too young to make a judgment, so whose judgment did you accept?

As you look back now with knowing eyes, were they right?

I recently met a teacher I'd known long ago, and we had not liked each other at all. We spent a very pleasant afternoon and found we had many interests in common, something I would never have suspected years before. When we were parting, he said, "I never knew you before today . . . you were in hiding." I was about to retort, "I wasn't *hiding* . . . you weren't *looking*." Then I realized we were both right. I *had* been hiding—and he *hadn't* been looking.

While you are trying to unearth yourself, ask yourself if you aren't trying to hide yourself lest people find out who you really are. And then wonder if who you really are isn't far more interesting than the camouflage you are wearing. At the same time, you might wonder if the images being offered by your family and friends are real. Or could they be surrounded by a shell of scars so thick and protective that they can't get out? It is said that *stone walls do not a prison make,* but we can build prisons for ourselves that can be opened only by magic, or by those we love.

The Gift of a Word, a Look, a Touch

You can hammer and pound on the thick, hardened overlay that surrounds the real selves of your loved ones with carping and criticism forever and it won't crack. But you *can* start a series of tiny chinks that will gradually run together and ultimately destroy it. Chinks in such armor are made with words, looks, and touch. Kind observations about others are gifts of great value. When I was in high school, I wanted to get into something known as the Chorus, a very exclusive singing group. I didn't think I could make it but I tried. I auditioned with Gounod's *Ave Maria,* which I had learned back in the convent. The lady with the "say" said she'd let me know. It was my first encounter with a form of

"Don't call us, we'll call you." I was pretty dejected when I stepped out into the hall. Standing quite close to the door were two of the school's cleaning ladies. "Was it yourself was singin' about the Blessed Lady?" I said yes, that it was. "Well, the angels couldn't have done better." I thanked them and went happily on my way. I didn't care if I made the Chorus or not, for somebody, I sang like an angel.

Now, you know they didn't have to say that. It would have been just as easy to have gone about their business; easier. After all, teenagers were unpredictable even then. But they had taken the trouble, and I was very grateful. As you can see, I never forgot it. Everyone does things right sometimes, so be on the watch for the opportunity to give the gift of a word. It is surely a gift that has great value, often far greater than the giver can know.

And what has this to do with sex? People with distorted self-images have a hard time opening up to love. They want to badly enough but they just don't know how to get past their own closed walls. There is a good deal of truth in the oft-said words that one must like oneself before it is possible to love others. When you feel good about yourself, everyone else seems pleasant or at least understandable. But where, when, and how do you start the job of peeling off other people's judgments?

Now is the time to begin, and here, in this room, is the place. Get a pencil and paper and start to make two lists. One is your credit list and the other your debit list. Under the credits, write down everything good you can think about yourself and then, under the debits, all the things that need fixing. When I first started this sort of personal accounting, I discovered some nice things about myself (I knew all the bad things). Then, instead of moaning about a sort of generalized situation labeled, "I'm a mess," a situation that paralyzes by its sheer enormity, you can compartmentalize it. You find out *what* really is a mess. Perhaps it's your overweight and, in particular, your protruding abdomen. A quick check with your Function Test back in the beginning of the book, which showed that you had difficulty with the Abdominal Strength Test, almost shouts the answer. Work to strengthen the abdominals, and the paunch will disappear . . . unless. The "unless" is to be found on your weight chart. If it shows you are really overweight and not just flabby, then a change in eating habits is indicated. If you have started to keep an Eat Sheet, you will be able to see exactly what you ate that contributed to that lumpy look and has probably also added dollops of fat to other places that might be even more crucial, like your heart. You know that unless you eat properly, exercise won't be enough. In order to look pleasing enough for others, and for yourself, the weight will have to come down.

While you *are* overweight, you aren't a hopeless mess either. Don't be blind to your good points. Everyone has attractive and not-so-attractive facets. There may be too much of you, but you stand well. Your shoulders may be droopy, but they are strong and wide. You might have a double chin, but your smile is genuine and your eyes are merry. Your weight may have slid down into your thighs, but your chest, arms, and waist are enviable. You have a chronic backache, but it doesn't show. You have a terrible swayback, but it never hurts. There really isn't anything that can't be improved once you know what it is you want to fix, and you fix your "debits" one by one. Probably, if you had a whole cluster of complaints (called a syndrome)—pain in your upper back, constant headaches, a stiff neck that makes desk work an agony, not to mention round shoulders and a concave chest—you'd be about ready to throw in the towel. The usual route would be aspirin for the headaches and backache (which could lead to stomach problems; aspirin is *not* harmless) and an analgesic for your neck. What should you start with? Well, what could cause headaches and a stiff neck? A round back could. And what causes a round back? Tight chest muscles and weak, overstretched upper-back muscles. So where do you begin? With exercises 12 and 14 to stretch the chest muscles, and exercises 3 and 66 to strengthen the back. Then you would add the fibrositis massage on page 174 to loosen up the tight tissue of the shoulders. You would do the shoulder shrugs often throughout your day, to prevent tension from undoing your good work. Pretty soon, as the tight chest gives up its hold on your shoulders and the upper back comes into its proper strength, your back and shoulders will straighten. The target area for tension would be kept so loose and relaxed that pain couldn't get in any licks and the headaches and stiff neck would just go away . . . and all because you straightened and strengthened your back. Overnight you will feel younger and more hopeful. Pretty soon you'd decide that if you aren't going to die right away you might as well live it up a little.

It's important to get rid of even the slightest pain that seems to linger more than a day or two, because pain can become chronic and can wreack havoc with your self-image. All of this might not be so important if that self-image didn't play such an almighty role in our lives. People who *know* they are healthy and attractive usually manage to convey that thought straight into the minds of others. Lucky are the children who are influenced to like and believe in themselves, for they become attractive children. Attractive children are treated differently from unattractive children, even by strangers. So are attractive adults. Attractive children view themselves in a rosy light, and they surround themselves with an aura of success and expectancy. This is carried over into adulthood, and since most of us get what we expect, they are given total acceptance.

Attractive people usually do well with sex; they attract it to themselves. They feel comfortable in situations involving their bodies and they take and give more satisfaction than do people who feel they are physically unattractive or who lack stamina and positive health.

The sad thing is that for many people, the sources of

their self-image feedback have been either in error or purposely destructive. In order to get an honest picture of the whole you, which you have been viewing for years only through other people's eyes, you may have to take it apart and look carefully at the pieces one by one, not as though they were parts of yourself, but just bits and pieces to be judged objectively. When you have looked at them carefully, judged them, and noted what should be improved on, put them back together and you will find a different you.

Make the following list in a notebook, carry it to your room, and forget all the preconceived notions about your appearance given to you by others and assimilated as gospel truth. "Remember, dear, never to wear green. Your skin is too sallow." Or, "Why in the world did you ever become a dancer? Look what it did to your legs." Or, "A fellow as short as you are should never wear checks, your father doesn't." Forget these things and, most important, forget the people who said them. *You* start now to judge for yourself. Look yourself over carefully and decide, not on the whole, but part by part, how you stack up.

Circle the adjectives that fit

Posture . . . straight, bent, sagging, sway-backed, round-backed, balanced, stiff, relaxed, flat-backed, forward head

Shoulders . . . broad, narrow, uneven, round, square, sagging, thin, fat, thick, weak, strong

Chest . . . broad, narrow, firm, saggy, well-muscled, fat

Breasts . . . firm, sagging, too much, not enough, flat, fat

Midriff . . . fat, thin, flabby, rolls, firm, smooth, tapering

Waist . . . small, average, thick, straight up and down, curves

Abdominals . . . flat, fat, firm, rounded, protruding, smooth

Hips . . . slender, tight, small, thin, fat, lumpy, smooth

Thighs . . . slender, smooth, well-muscled, fat, fibrositic, lumpy, soft, hard

Knees . . . strong, weak, bony, fat, damaged
Calves . . . slender, rounded, well-muscled, smooth, lumpy, thin, thick
Ankles . . . slender, heavy, strong, weak, swollen, thick, fat, thin
Feet . . . strong, weak, flat, high arch, smooth, calloused, long second toe, bunions, flexible, tight
Legs . . . strong, weak, slender, fat, fibrositic, varicosed, curved, bony, well-muscled
Back . . . straight, arched, rounded, flat, strong, weak, painful, thin, fat, sagging, bent, well-muscled
Arms . . . fat, thin, strong, weak, smooth, lumpy, well-muscled, flabby
Skin . . . smooth, firm, slightly wrinkled, very wrinkled, clear, saggy, tight, good color, sallow, tan, broken out
Face . . . handsome, beautiful, attractive, cheerful, pleasant, gloomy, severe, merry, sad, kind, unpleasant, morose

There may be other adjectives you will want to apply, and there may be other parts of yourself that you will want to include. Just be sure you don't leave out anything you consider important, either as a plus or a minus. In the chapter on "Pain—Preserver of Sexuality," you will be given a chance to list what hurts, what once hurt and therefore may again, if you don't take preventive measures.

Abdominals

The protruding abdomen on either male or female *at any age* is a disaster area. The bigger it is, the greater is the disaster. You can, of course, hide it (sort of) under a loose shirt or mu-mu. However, even if the wind doesn't blow shirt or skirt against your protuberant belly—say it, *protuberant belly*—and even if you don't have to dance cheek to cheek, *you* keep bumping into it all day long. *You* know it's there when you undress at night and when you cover it as best you can in the morning, and *you* feel it bouncing like a basketball in a bag of old clothes when you run for the bus. And you don't have to be fat to have the problem. A "pot" can be caused by abdominal weakness and is quite as loud an advertisement of inadequacy as the balloon belly.

Whether you are fat or slim, male or female, young or old, if you have abdominal weakness you are asking for trouble. And you can't live up to your lovemaking potential even if you were to spend four hours a day with "how-to" manuals. To strengthen and flatten, use exercises 1, 2, and 8 *many times a day*. Measure and measure so that you are constantly aware of the problem as well as the cure. If you do the exercises the problem will disappear, unless, of course, you are obese. That will call for a change in eating habits. The combination will most assuredly work. If you go slowly and surely, fat will disappear. If you have been really outsize, you may be left with a problem, an apron of empty flesh hanging down from the base of the abdomen, and there's no way to roll it up and stick a pin in it. Plastic surgery, on the advice of a competent physician, is a possibility. The operation for the removal of the hanging apron is called abdominoplasty and it is certainly worth the bother, if greater sexuality is one of your aims. The girl with no bust in her bra cannot be filled with any more apprehension concerning tactile discovery than the person with an empty old pocket where her flat stomach should be.

Before you consider the extreme measure of plastic surgery, spend as long as it takes to get your weight down to what is right for your frame and build. No plastic surgeon in the world is going to slim you down by cutting away unwanted fat. You only see that in the movies. You will have to do the work of getting rid of it naturally, and you will have to improve your abdominal muscles naturally too, with the exercises. *Then* see the surgeon, if you still have to.

In order to hurry the fat on its way, use the fibrositis massage described a little further on. While the abdomen is not a target area for tension and thickened tissue, it does respond when fat is made uncomfortable with kneading and pinching.

Ankles

Ankles can be too thin or too thick, and they can be either weak or inflexible. If they are either thin or weak, the same exercises will strengthen and fill them out with muscle. Use exercises 11, 13, and 62. If the ankle is inflexible (you found out in test 14 for the soleus), spend a great deal of time on this exercise. You can do it on curbstones and stairs, stepping on a book or off the edge of the porch.

If you are not generally obese but do have thick ankles, you can be fairly certain that you tense them when you are under pressure and have developed fibrositis. The massage will help to speed the thickening away. Pinch and knead up toward the heart and *then* do your exercises.

Arms

Upper arms, when they are lacking in muscle, look puny and weak—because they are. If they are the target areas for tension, they will look lumpy even though thin. If they are tension targets and also fat, they will be hard and resisting. *That stuff is not muscle.* Muscle, when it is in good condition and not buried in fibrositis, is soft and pliable unless you contract it. Then it becomes hard and smooth. To improve strength and to get rid of fat, use exercise 7, and exercises 12 and 14 with weight bags in your hands. Numbers 24 and 34 will help too. Use the push-ups (page 30) and chin-ups (page 31). At least three times a week, do the weight training exercises 63–65. If you have fibrositis, use the massage *before* you exercise. Do exercise 16 every time you wash your hands. Incidentally, if you are female, don't worry about becoming *muscular*. The muscle will be there, but you won't *see* it except in your improved figure, tennis game, swim stroke, and total comfort in sleeveless shirts.

Back

Your back, any and all of it, is of the greatest importance. If it is weak, it can make your days and nights miserable. It can prevent you from doing your best work, from enjoying sports and vacations, driving your car, sleeping, and making love. There are several problems to be found in backs, but by far the most damaging are tension and inflexibility. When back problems are discussed, they are often diagnosed as "arthritis," or "discs." Actually, only 20 percent of the back troubles serious enough to need clinical care are pathological. Eighty percent are due to muscle deficiency and can be corrected with *the right exercise*. It is quite true that X-rays have revealed "arthritis" and "discs" that seemed to be causing the trouble. But too often, after the "disc" was removed, the trouble continued. And many is the strong back that had "arthritis" but suffered not a twinge of pain. To be safe, see to it that your back remains both strong and flexible. If you failed test 6 back in the beginning of the book, you aren't flexible. If you failed either test 4 or 5, your back isn't strong either. If you failed tests 1 and/or 2 *and* 6, you probably already have a backache.

The Limbering Series, Exercises 73–76

If you have a back that gives you *any* trouble at all, do the following exercises every morning before you get out of bed and every evening before you get in. If you begin to feel twinges anywhere along its length, add two more back-exercise series during the day, midmorning and midafternoon. If you are under pressure (any kind, from trying to get a promotion to handling a difficult domestic problem) and your back kicks up, remember that it didn't come from sitting in a draft. It came either from weakness or from inflexibility, *plus tension.*

If you have had a back episode severe enough to send you to the doctor, take this book to him and show him the exercises and ask him for a prescription for a coolant spray to interrupt spasm. Coaches and doctors used to use a chemical called ethyl chloride for this purpose, but it was explosive, very cold, and could be used as an anesthetic. With those properties, it wasn't released to the public. But the new spray is not explosive, won't freeze your skin, and is about as useful as an anesthetic as cleaning fluid. However, when sprayed along a painful muscle as you stretch that muscle, it will interrupt the impulse that is causing the muscle to react to its pain with spasm, which alas, causes even more pain and therefore more spasm.

73. Supine Knee-to-Nose and Stretch

Lie supine with knees bent and feet about six inches apart. Raise your head and try to bring your right knee in to touch your nose. Lie back down as you extend the leg forward to a point about ten inches from the floor. Return it to the knee-bent resting position. Do the same with the left leg and alternate legs, four to each side. Roll over onto your left side.

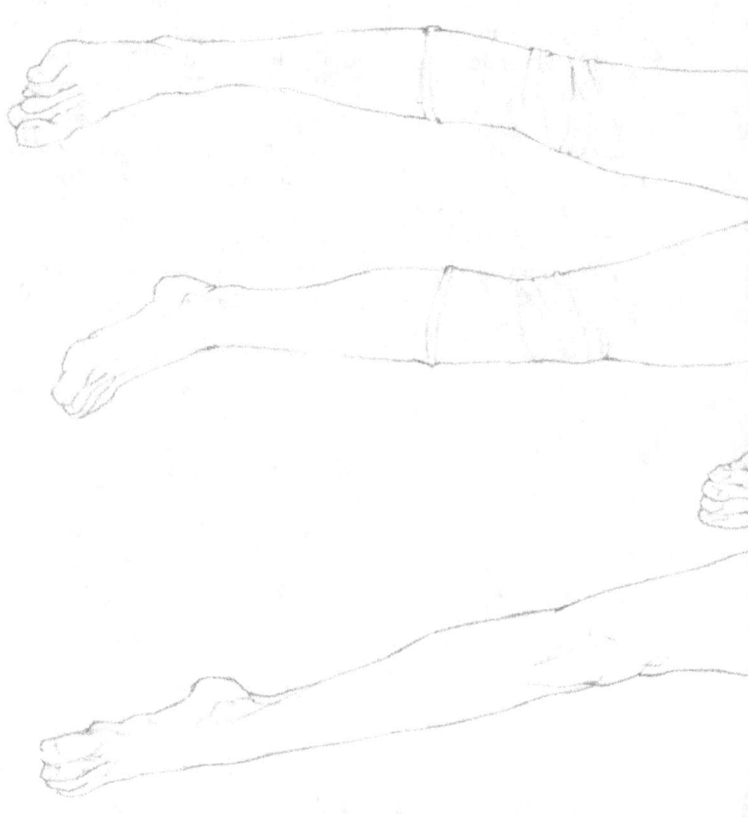

74. Side-Lying Knee-to-Chest and Extend

(This is the time to use the spray.) Rest your head on your left arm, bring your right knee to your chest then extend it straight down to a point parallel with the left leg and about ten inches above it. Lower *and relax*.

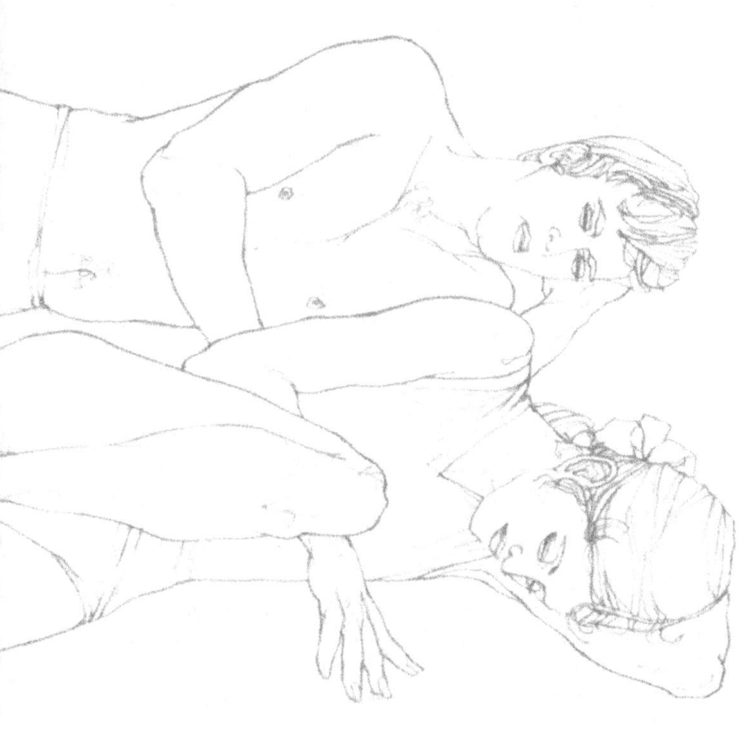

Remember, there is rarely a backache without tension. Don't hurry through these or you will build more tension. *Relax.* Do four of these knee-to-chest movements and then roll to the prone position with head resting on your arms.

75. Prone Pelvic Tilt or Gluteal Set

Pinch the buttocks tight together, and as you hold tight, pull in your abdominals. Hold the double contraction for a slow count of four and release. Relax completely and repeat. Do four and then roll over onto your right side.

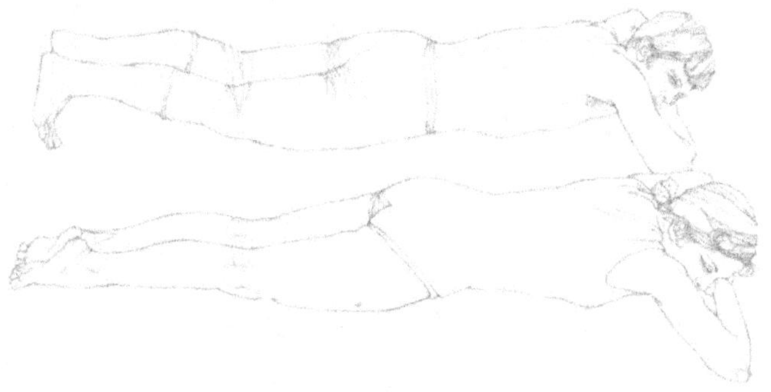

Repeat exercise 74, *side-lying knee-to-chest and extend,* four times with the left leg. This is another chance to spray. Have the person doing the exercise *point* to the painful spot, and then, as the exercise is performed, spray all along the muscle. Remember, you are just trying to interrupt an impulse, not freeze a muscle. If the spray is going to be able to help, it will help at once. Two or three repetitions of the exercise will be enough to tell you. Ask the person where it hurts now. The answer will either be a surprised, "Why it doesn't hurt at all," or, "I can't quite tell." In the first case, do a few more of the exercises. In the latter, ask him or her to *point* to the spot if possible. Often the answer will be that it hurts in the same place but the pointing will be to an entirely different place. That's an excellent sign. The spasms are giving up the ghost one by one; you've knocked out one and have uncovered a second.

(The above system works on many muscles, from sprained ankles to shoulders with "bursitis," "tennis elbows," stiff necks, and even tension-caused headaches.)

76. Supine Bent-Knee Pelvic Tilt

Roll again onto your back, which brings you around full circle. Bend your knees with feet slightly apart as before. Arch the back so that a mouse might sit under the arch. Keep both seat and shoulders flat on the floor. Now, press your back down hard and flatten the mouse. Hold the pelvic tilt for a slow count of four. Relax and repeat. Do four. That completes one round. You should really do two rounds to be sure of protection.

Check your mattress. A soft one is often the cause of morning stiffness. If you have to travel a lot, ask for a firm mattress. If you get a soft one, toss the mattress on the floor. It will work just fine. Incidentally, you shouldn't make love on a soft bed either. Or a squeaky one (but that's another matter). In either case, the floor is always there.

If your back is tight, (you have only to check your results in tests 6 and 13 to know if it is) do the flexibility bounces, exercise 5, *often*. Keep in mind that tension is contributing to your back tightness, and tension is all the time. Try using the penny system to remind you throughout the day to do this exercise.

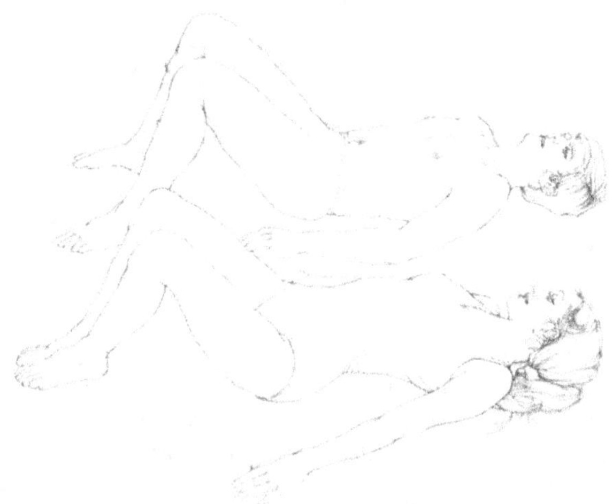

Back Fibrositis

The thickness that shows up on tight shoulders, hips, thighs, arms, back of neck, and knees is more fond of the back than almost anywhere else. It can settle anywhere. Read the next section on Fibrositis Massage carefully and be sure to add it to your program.

Fibrositis Massage

To begin with, fibrositis massage isn't pleasant, it isn't relaxing, and at first it hurts. If your circulation is poor, you may bruise. *But it does work.* There are some places where you can do it for yourself, namely the thighs, knees, and upper arms. However, when it comes to the backs and sides of the upper legs, the dowager's hump on the back of the neck, the shoulders, back, and hips, you will need help.

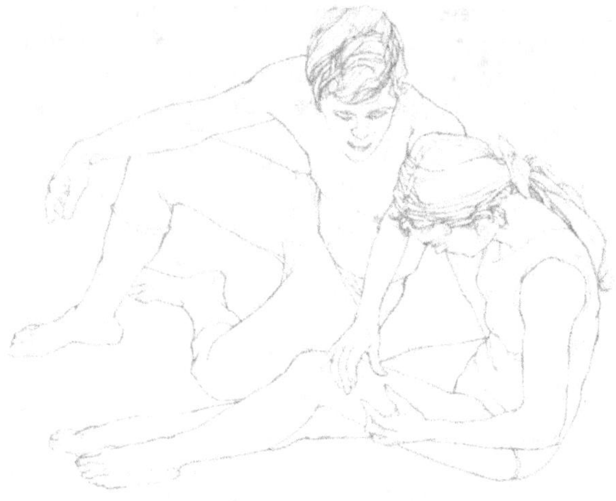

Thighs. Sit with relaxed legs (and an egg timer—three minutes to any one area is enough). Take both hands to the same thigh, and working toward your heart, knead, twist, roll, and use any other action you can dream up to break up the thickened tissue. If you use TV commercials to time your massage, you can cover a lot of ground in an evening. Always smooth the worked area with strong hand pressure toward the heart after churning it up. Think that you have pulled a lot of unwanted material loose and your smoothing hands are sending it up to some sort of clearing house for removal. Then get up and do the exercise that the area requires. Thighs need deep knee bends and exercises 28, 29, 30, and 35.

Arms. Reach around to the back of your left elbow with your right hand and press your left lower arm across your waist. Start working up the back of the arm, kneading all the way up to your shoulder. Start again at the elbow, kneading the side of your arm that faces straight forward when your lower arm is against your waist. That's the prime target area for tension in the arm. Work your way up to the shoulder. Next, drop your arm so that the back of your hand rests against your thigh. Knead the tissue over the biceps right up into and over the shoulder to its outermost point. Repeat these kneadings three times. Yes, it hurts . . . it has to hurt . . . and it will hurt less as you soften it up. If you should bruise when you start this and before your circulation improves, think nothing of it. If someone asks "Good heavens! How did you get those finger bruises on your arms?" Look smug and say something like, "You wouldn't believe me if I told you," and let it go at that.

When you have finished your arm massage, do exercise 16 immediately, and don't forget to smooth the area with firm hand pressure toward the heart. Do the other exercises that will improve the arms.

Knees. There are two spots that tension uses as targets in the knees: one is just below the kneecap to the inside of the leg, and the other is just below the kneecap and to the outside toward the back. Use the same system of kneading, smoothing, and pushing toward the heart, and then do *deep knee bends.*

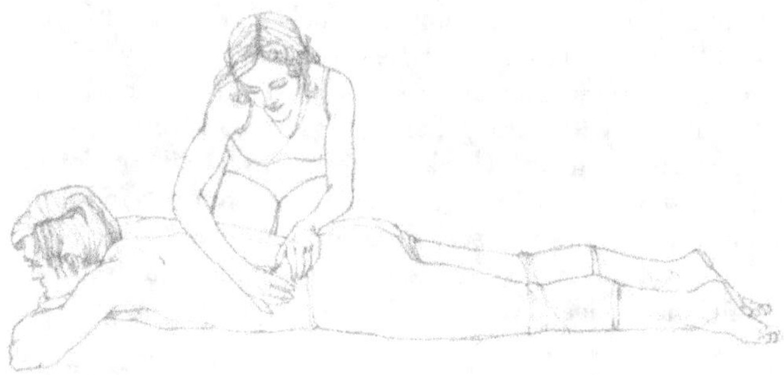

Back. Here is where you will need help. Pinch and knead the thickened, tender tissue, wherever you can find it, all the way up the back. Smooth and then do exercise 5, the flexibility bounces, and the prone arm lifts in exercise 26. Finish up with exercise 8.

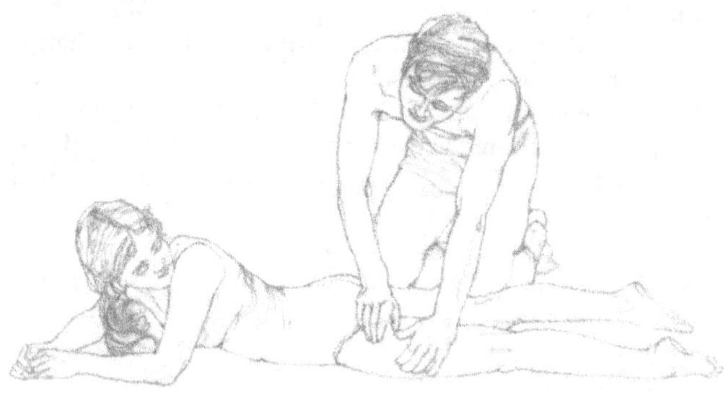

Hips. If there is thickness to the sides of the hips, an area called "saddlebags," this calls for grasping great gobs of the fatty tissue and squeezing as you knead. This area, like the others, will be exquisitely tender. Give about a minute's workout to each side, smooth, and then do exercises 19, 21, and 71.

Shoulders. Of them all, the shoulders are the worst tension targets. Have the "sufferer" lie prone or sit with relaxed arms. Start kneading at the point of the shoulder

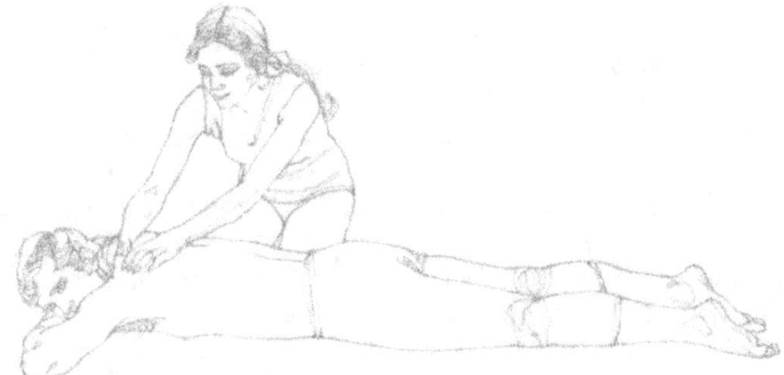

and work up the neck into the hairline. This area hurts the most, so be comparatively gentle at first. In two weeks you will be able to attack with much more force. Smooth and do exercise 14 and add shoulder shrugs.

77. Shoulder Shrugs

Pull your shoulders up to your ears and hold for three seconds. Then press your shoulders down to make a long neck. Hold for three seconds. Round your shoulders forward, touching the backs of your hands together. Hold for three seconds. Finally, press your shoulders back as though you were trying to make your elbows touch. Hold for three seconds, then shake them loose. Don't wait until your shoulders start to ache to do this exercise. Find things that happen all day that you can tie it into—answering the phone, changing chores, changing the paper in your typewriter, getting something from the files—anything will do, just so long as the shrug series goes on intermittently all day long.

Back

Now, back to *backs* and the other problems they suffer. The one most easily noticed is the *round back.* The one seen most often on girls and women is the *swayback,* and the one nobody pays much attention to is the *flat back.*

Round back. It is caused when the chest muscles foreshorten and the upper back muscles are overstretched. Do exercises 12, 14, and 66.

Swayback. It is seen when the pelvis tips back too far to cause a deep curve in the lower back, forcing the hips out. Do exercises 1, 2, and one-half of 43, the cat back or pelvic tilt on all fours. Push up into the angry-cat position, but when you lower, don't go into the full down-arch. Stop when your back is level.

Flat back. The flat back looks like a flat back. It is the opposite of the swayback and has too little curve at the waist. Do exercise 43 (with emphasis on the downward arch), and all the pelvic tilts, 37 through 45.

Breasts

Breasts are lovely things, and we begin to appreciate them from our first hours in the world. Through them comes the food which we need for life, and behind them dwells the reassuring beating heart that filled Paradise Lost. If a young mother is handed her baby anytime within the first twenty-four hours of its birth, she will unerringly place its head against her left breast, even if she is left-handed. It seems she too is programmed with certain information. The breast continues to remain a symbol of comfort, sustenance, and sexuality. In America this is often carried to extremes, and the girl who is sparsely endowed has been made to feel unfeminine, as if that's where femininity resided! The girl who is overly provided is just as miserable, and many a foolish emotional hang-up hangs on a pound of flesh.

One of the problems is that the breast develops (or doesn't) at an age when girls are so concerned about their appearance that any departure from what is considered desirable seems as noticeable as a wart on the end of the nose. If the young girl is really flat-chested, she can disguise the "disgraceful" lack under padded bras, but she lives in terror of the time when a boy may slide a searching hand under that fluffy fraud and discover what? Nothing!

If the girl develops and develops until she has a bosom like a front porch, she's in even bigger trouble. Should she be obese, diet and exercise *may* help, but there is no guarantee. Outsize breasts are often seen on very slender, even fragile-looking girls. The problem is called hypertrophy of the breast, and quite apart from the damage to her psyche (kids are never reticent when it comes to giving out such nicknames as "cow" or "milk shake"), she may have to lean back to support that balustrade, causing her back to sway. She may become round-backed instead. Deep grooves appear in her shoulders from straps supporting the weight, and her chest cannot expand properly. This means that her lungs cannot be well aerated and her chest wall becomes rigid from lack of motion. As if these miseries were not enough, many surgeons consider such breasts an invitation to cancer. The answer to this particular problem seems to be plastic surgery, and the sooner the better. The operation is called reduction mammoplasty, and since it exists, there isn't a reason in the world to endure such misery and humiliation. If the operation is done early enough, both lactation and nipple sensation remain intact.

At the other extreme, the person with a chest too flat for happy self-acceptance can undergo a corrective operation known as augmentation mammoplasty. This was once considered a dangerous operation, but in 1963 Dr. Frank Gerow and Dr. Thomas Cronin started to use a new material developed by Dow Chemical Company called Silastic, or silicone. Augmentation mammoplasty is managed in some cases by affixing a gel implant (a seamless implant filled with a gel and shaped like a teardrop) to the chest wall behind the breast tissue. The result is a normal-looking breast which also *feels* like a breast and responds to stimulation as a breast should. If the owner of such implants has a baby, she can lactate normally and the baby can be breast-fed, which should happen if at all possible—for the sake of both the baby and the mother.

There is an even newer twist to be found here and there across the country. It is an inflatable implant consisting of a bladder of silicone rubber which can be introduced through a very small opening under the breast and then filled with a saline solution, or dextran, a heavy molecular sugar. It can be inflated to any desired size and is of especial value when breast sizes are unequal. This implant is even softer than the Dow implant and continues to remain soft over the years. If, through accident, the bladder should rupture, the contents are easily absorbed by the body and a new bladder can be implanted at the site of the old scar.

Then there is a condition that usually happens to older women, but not always; it is a *ptosed* or "dropped" breast. This happens when the skin has become distended with time or after tremendous weight loss. Then an operation called masopexy can be performed. In this case, the surgeon's job is to cut away the stretched skin, resculpture the breast into a well-fitting "brassiere," and reposition both nipple and aureole. There will of course be some scarring—a curved scar under the breast and a straight-line scar downward from nipple to the curved scar. However, a scar is a little thing compared to a saggy, baggy breast, and it can be covered very nicely with a bra, a nightie, or some makeup.

Needless to say, you don't cart your bosom to a plastic surgeon without first trying every home remedy in the book. If you want to *augment* your breast size, use the weight series, exercises 67, 68, and 69. Those exercises will build muscle; that's what makes weight lifters look as if they need a size 38D. The muscle *under* the breast grows and pushes what breast you have up and out. If you need *reduction,* and the rest of you needs reduction as well, it is certainly worth a try. No matter what you want to do, if you are obese, lose weight first.

Chest

The male chest that has run to fat often looks exactly like what a female might pay over one thousand dollars to have added to her own chest wall. In short, he has a bust line where his chest line should be. The first step, of course, is diet and exercise. Start with push-ups and go on to exercises 12, 18, 22, 24, 34, and 63 through 69. If weight loss, increased strength, and muscle build-up don't quite take up the slack, then a plastic surgeon certainly can. In this case, it is with little more than a few tucks. But tucks are at best an emergency treatment. The best answer is to remain (or become) slim, hard, and healthy. That's going to take work, but what a joy to feel wonderful and to look wonderful, not only to everyone else, *but to yourself.*

If the male chest is skinny and narrow, it's ten to one that the rest of the body is of the same general appearance. That calls for weight training and lots of it. Use the breathing exercises in the section on relaxation to increase your lung and chest size. Use the running exercises to demand that your lungs work fully. Don't forget to use plenty of stretch (flexibility) exercises to keep your muscles loose and free of tension.

It should be kept in mind that while sex is of tremendous importance to man's happiness, there *are* other things. A fine body can also be used on the ski slopes, high in the mountains, on a tennis court, in fact in all those places where sexuality is only thinly disguised by action all day—and leads without a break in rhythm to lovemaking at night. There's nothing that says you have to wait until after dark, either!

Calves

Skinny calves are not an asset, nor are weak calf muscles or thick, heavy lower legs. If your lower legs are not adding anything to your self-image, you can

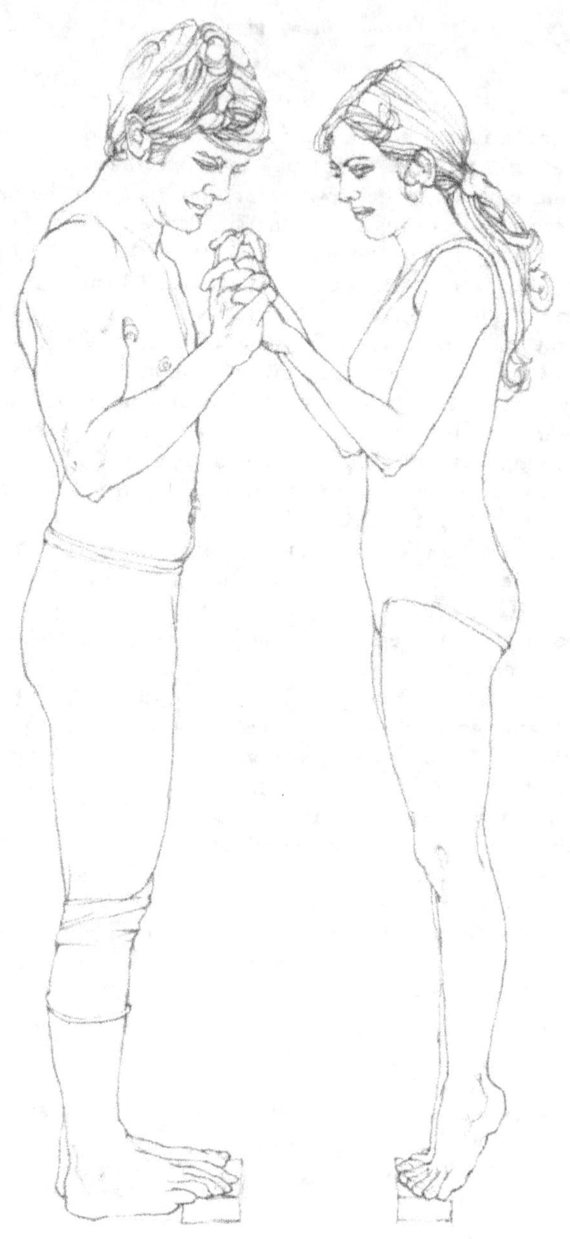

change them. To strengthen (and therefore fill out), use exercise 78. Add all the runs, plus exercises 11 and 13.

If your lower legs are heavy and the rest of you is not, use the fibrositis massage described on page 174.

78. Toe Raises

Stand with the soles of your feet resting on a brick, block of wood, or the edge of a stair. Let your heels rest on the floor or, as in the case of the stair, hanging down free in the air. This position stretches the soleus, or heel cords. Now rise to full toe stand (also include exercises 11 and 13 so you can get higher on your toes) and lower. As foot strength and lower-leg strength improve, hang weight bags on your shoulders, or wear a pack with an ever-increasing weight load, or carry two weighted suitcases, one in each hand. Start with eight raises and work up to fifty. Then start adding weight.

Face

There are a great many facial products and exercises offered yearly on the market, and the usual promise made is that if you do those exercises, use that cream, or get the suggested facial and plaster yourself with mud, your skin will be seamless and smooth. Not so. Your face is you, and to keep it as smooth as a baby's behind (or your own) really shouldn't be your aim in life. There's nothing against keeping it attractive, but lots of attractive faces have a few wrinkles. It's the direction those lines take that counts. If you are down and sad and unhappy most of the time, the lines are going to look down, sad, and unhappy. If you are happy with yourself and those around you, they are going to add to your looks.

The tone of your facial muscles and skin do matter, and neither can be controlled with mud, cream, or facial exercise. They depend on the food you eat, your circulation, and general level of fitness. Creams, facials, and makeup enhance a face. But instead of real general conditioning? No way. Get your whole body in shape, and unless too many years, too much sorrow, or too many bad eating habits have damaged your face past the point of recall by moderate means, you will improve your face too. If you can't, there's always plastic surgery. Plastic surgery can indeed roll the years back but it can't make you twenty-one, so don't expect it. The time it makes sense to have it done is when you have put your body into great shape and need a face and neck to go with it. It is usually done after the whole edifice is in a shambles. That's exactly like putting a brand new shiny door on a deteriorating tenement house where the furnace has been carted off by vandals and all the water pipes froze and broke last winter.

Many people whose livelihood depends on a youthful appearance have plastic surgery. They have hair transplants and spend many hours a week exercising their bodies. They also eat sparingly and properly. If you need plastic surgery, or think you do, then go about it the right and lasting way. *Get in total physical shape first and then go ahead.* Before the day you are scheduled for that surgery, however, see to it that your whole body is slender, strong, and flexible. Topping it off with a face that has fewer wrinkles and sags will then make good sense.

Feet

Feet are very important to your self-image. They make the difference when it comes to the way you walk. If your feet are weak, you will paddle along. And who ever dreamed of a paddling romantic? If your feet are inflexible, you will stalk—and that's not too romantic either. If you clomp, waddle, or flap when you run, you can count on being left out of the neighborhood game of "touch," and your efforts on the tennis court won't get you a second invitation. Nobody has yet found the fountain of youth, but anyone with lousy feet knows the quickest way to old age.

79. Inward Rotation

Flat feet. If you have them, you have them, and that's that. But you can make them work just as well and as painlessly as the kind with built-in arches. Strengthen the *anterior tibialis,* the muscle running down the outside of the lower leg, over the instep and, like a stirrup, running *under* your arch. Sit with legs stretched out in front and turn your toes in and then pull them up toward your body. Hold for a slow count of four. Relax and repeat. Do them whenever there is a commercial on TV.

Long second toe. That's hereditary, and it isn't nice. A good foot catches your weight on the heel and throws it forward onto two points, the big-toe joint in the ball of the foot, and the outside of the foot near the little toe. The foot with a long second toe (called "the classic Greek foot" after all those models for Greek sculptors) does not act that way. The second-toe joint in the ball of the foot is right in the middle, so your weight moves forward from the heel to the center of the foot, as though you were on a tightrope. You are under constant strain to keep your balance, and the joints of the ankles, knees, and hips often wear unevenly, like tires on poorly balanced wheels. A callus appears in the center of the ball of the foot where the second-toe joint is striking. A second one grows on the outside of the big toe, and a third on the outside of the foot near the little toe. Sooner or later the big toe starts to turn inward and can then present you with a bunion. Callused, corny, bunioned feet are unsexy and unnecessary. To help this situation wear a quarter-inch felt pad, three-quarter-inch diameter, in your shoes just under the first joint of your big toe *in the ball of your foot.* Or use the kind you can stick onto the foot itself. Go barefoot as often as you can, and strengthen your feet and ankles (toe raises) and knees (knee bends). Use the following "walks" whenever you are puttering about the house and the music that pleases you comes on the radio. (Nothing says you can't do them deliberately to the records or tapes of your choice!)

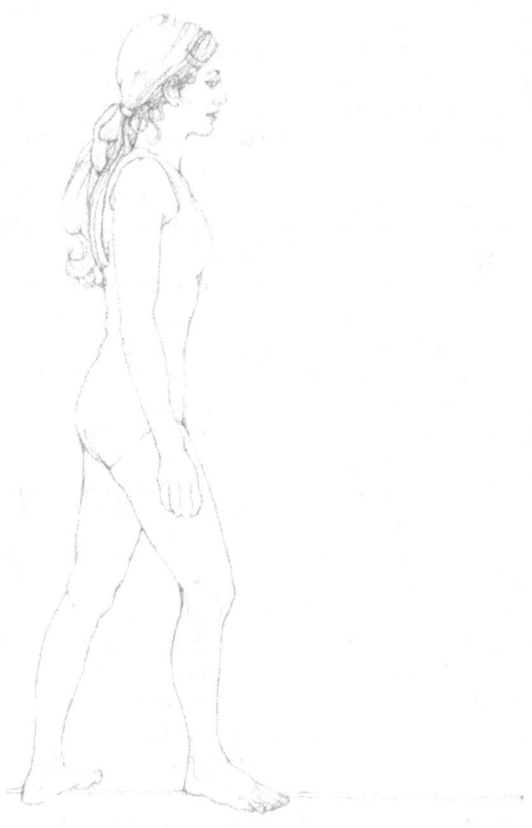

80. Turned-out Walk

Corrects pigeon toes and clumsy gait

Run a strip of tape down the hall, across the kitchen, or use the cracks between the boards in the floor as guides. Walk forward and backward on the tape with toes turned way out. Do the steps in an easy walking posture, then with knees bent, and finally with legs stiff, as though your knees are encased in plaster. Do this exercise often, and you will find your walk improving even if you don't have obvious problems such as pigeon toes.

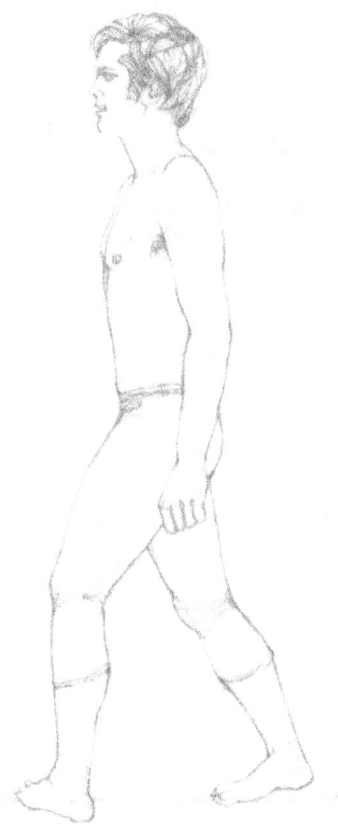

81. Turned-in Walk

This helps with feet that have a way of pointing out

If you walk along with feet turned way out, there is a good chance that you have flat feet, and a swayback to boot. Train your feet to track straight ahead by overemphasizing the turn *in*. This also strengthens the *anterior tibialis* for flat feet and, oddly enough, reduces the "saddlebags" on the sides of the hips.

82. Toe Bounces

Walk along on your toes, coming down to your heel and going all the way up with each step. The lift should be so high as to *almost* lift you off the floor into a skip. When your feet feel like taking off, clear the floor by less than an inch at first. Later go higher until you are up into a skip. This strengthens all the muscles in the feet.

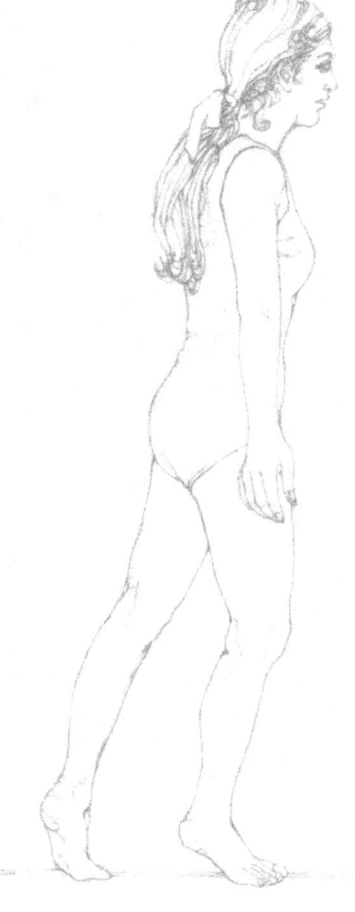

Hands

Hands should be strengthened, and they should be cared for (like feet). Ugly broken nails, dry, rough skin, and hard calluses just don't add up to sensitive sexuality. It's amazing how much time, effort, and money a man will spend on his beard and hair; and then even forget to *wash* his hands and feet. It is even more amazing to note the care given to outer trappings by women who forget to remove cracked nail polish from fingers and toes.

To strengthen your hands, keep a ball near your telephone. Whenever you talk, squeeze the ball with first one hand and then the other. There is nothing like a fishy handshake to turn off the formation of a romantic bond.

Hips

Hips can make or break the figure. When one thinks of sex, it is impossible to ignore hips. When they are soft and flabby, the sex act is influenced by those two very descriptive words. They add up to "What am I doing here?"

Use exercises 4, 17, 19, 21, 24–29, 37–46, 61, 62, and 71.

Use the fibrositis massage on page 174 to reduce the size of your hips, and always remember that the man or woman with the tight seat at least *looks* as though he or she knows what it's all about.

Knees

Fat knees can be slimmed by attention to diet, the exercises that strengthen them, and by fibrositis massage. Weak knees and damaged knees need strengthening, and the surest way to strengthen knees is with deep knee bends. If you came up through the schools in the last twenty years, you were probably blessed with the totally erroneous information that nobody should do full knee bends because they caused damage to the miniscus (cartilage). That is not what caused the knee injuries that led to that idiotic conclusion. The game of football, which does damage knees, caused that conclusion when several players developed torn cartilages doing something called the duck walk. One would ask why Austrian skiers don't suffer similarly when doing duck walks, nor do Russian gymnasts or Scandinavian distance runners. Why only to American football players, and occasionally a weight lifter (who most probably played football in high school)? The reason is clear. Americans (even athletes) don't walk very much, and *legs are built by walking when you are very young.* We have that particular injury in such profusion because we don't build children's legs when they're still young and we don't give our high-school players enough conditioning before the season. If you want strong knees, do knee bends, climb stairs, run cross-country, ski cross-country, hike hills, and carry a pack. Add the following exercise to your walk series.

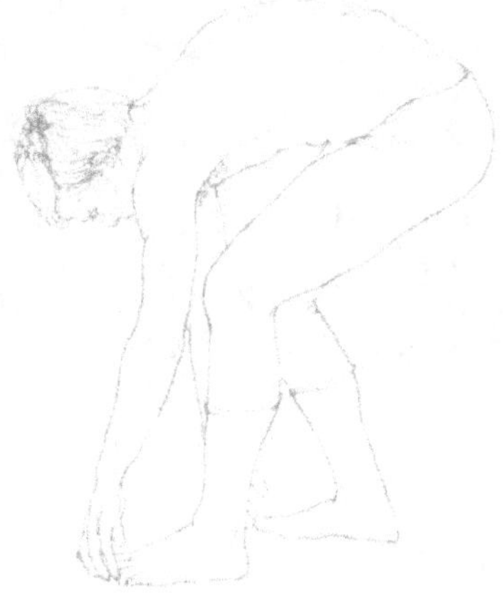

83. Bent Walk

Bend your knees and bend over forward so that your fingers can drag along the floor. Lead with your heels as you progress across the floor. Keep your feet facing forward.

Legs

To strengthen, do exercises 9, 11, 13, 15, 19, 21, 25–30, 35, 42, 44, 70, 71, and 78–82.

For flexibility, do exercises 5, 17, 47, 48, 53, and 55.

To slim, use the fibrositis massage.

There is a condition that attacks the legs and the self-image at the same time, varicose veins. They are hereditary, so if your parents suffered from them, you can be almost certain to find those ugly blue tracings on your own legs some day. However, there is much that can be done to hold them off (and hold them in).

Varicose veins appear when the veins lose their elasticity and the tiny valves along their length fail to operate efficiently. When that happens, they don't close properly, and backflow takes place. This further swells the veins, and they begin to break down. Usually, women first encounter this problem when they are pregnant and the pressure of the growing fetus is added to that created by gravity. Both men and women with the tendency toward varicosity will hasten its appearance when their occupations demand either long hours of standing (not walking) and/or sitting. Standing causes the blood to pool in the legs, and sitting does the same thing and compresses the circulatory system in thighs and hips as well. Both cause muscle to lose tone. The elastic stockings people wear for varicose veins only add insult to injury, for they not only do nothing at all to remedy the situation, but further complicate the condition by interfering with circulation. What's the prognosis? The veins continue to break down, more appear, and aching begins. When the condition becomes bad enough, a surgeon is engaged to "strip" the worst of the malfunctioning veins, and the remaining veins then take over their work. Given time and the same conditions, those too will break down into ugly meandering, sluggish streams. What is needed of course is a change in the conditions surrounding the weakness.

The very best support hose for veins are muscles that

are in excellent condition and used constantly as aids to the heart pump in its endeavors to get the blood up into the body and back to itself. The single best exercise for this purpose is again the deep knee bend. Knee bends strengthen the muscles themselves, and when the legs are in the bending position they squeeze the blood along its way. It should be obvious that ten knee bends done before breakfast are not going to help much if you have to stand at a control panel, ironing board, blackboard, or next to a dentist's chair for three hours before lunch. They won't help much if your morning will be spent sitting in a car or at a desk. What will be needed are several knee bends, done intermittently throughout the day, plus such assists as climbing stairs and a brisk walk or two. If you are at home, you can use the tenpenny system. The shopkeeper can "look for something" under the counter or in the stockroom at the close of each sale. The dentist "needs something" in the bottom drawer after each patient has departed.

In addition to those ongoing exercises that must become a part of *every* day, keep your legs up on the desk, table, footstool or railing whenever you can, and use the following exercises in your program: 11, 13, 15, 19, 21, 25, 26, 28–31, 33, 35, 36, 57–59, 61, 62, 70, 71, and 79–83.

Midriff

As a general exercise program goes into effect and sensible eating habits are observed, the extra weight padding the torso will begin to disappear. The exercises will build the attractive and very necessary muscles in this area. The special exercises which develop this area for your sexual pleasure are, first, the waist twists, exercise 8. They need to be done many times a day, and the best way to assure remembering to do them is by using ten pennies and a cup. Put ten pennies next to a cup in your bathroom and start your day with one full glass of water. Each time you use the bathroom, do your selected exercises (which usually include the waist twists, deep knee bends, and flexibility bounces (exercise 5) and take less than a minute and a half), drop one penny in the cup and drink a glass of water. The glass of water will get you back in there again, and again, and again. It will also help your body in its weight-reduction program.

If you work at an office and can't possibly leave ten pennies around in the bathroom, put them in one pocket and move them to another as you complete your selected exercise. If someone comes in and catches you bending, bouncing, or twisting and asks what you are doing, just answer "Sexercises; the book's in a plain wrapper in my bottom desk drawer." You *know* nobody's going to think you are strange after that.

The other midriff exercises are 10, 16, 17, 20, 22, 23, 25, 31, 34, 38, 41, 42, 43, 44, 46, and 49.

Posture

Posture is made up of many facets, and you contribute to yours by the physical condition of your body, past habits of movement, and by what you *permit* your various and varying emotional states to do to you. You could work for months to stretch tight chest muscles and strengthen overstretched and weakened upper back muscles (the prime causes of a rounded back), and then, the first time your life takes a swoop downward you could undo the whole thing by hunching over in defeat. *Know* how your body reacts to problems and consciously prevent that destructive reaction. Increased strength and flexibility, plus awareness of any posture anomaly you may have developed over the years, can build a better posture. But only your mind can maintain it.

Shoulders

To strengthen shoulders and increase their breadth (if only through increased muscle size), do push-ups and chin-ups. For increased strength, do exercises 18,

22, and 24. Use weight bags when you do 7, 10, 12, 14, and 16. Use the weight-training series, 63–69. To loosen and stretch, use the following without weights: 7, 10, 12, 14, 16, 23, 26, 34, and 77.

Keep in mind that shoulders are a prime target area for tension and if that's where tension affects you, be sure to use the shoulder shrugs, exercise 77, often every day and try to get someone else to do the pinching massage on you every evening. This is also a problem that one of those mechanical belts will help. Contrary to the usual belief, they will not slim you; however, they can loosen tight, thickened tissue which has formed over and around muscles.

Thighs

Thighs, second only to shoulders as tension target areas, need massage if they are thick, dimpled, and painful when pinched. They also need knee bends many times a day, but don't be too ambitious when you start them. Use the ten-penny system and do two deep knee bends each time you go into the bathroom. *Only two.* Keep that going for a full week even if you know you can do at least a dozen. The second week, add two more. It isn't the number you can do that counts, *it's the habit of doing some every time you enter that room* that's going to count from then on. Doing two or four doesn't seem an unsurmountable task even if you have no exercise habits as yet. If you undertook doing twelve to start out, you might be in a hurry once or twice and omit them altogether. That would be the beginning of habit disintegration. By the time you've been doing them *every time* for a month, you will feel something is terribly wrong if you quit or even simply skip a session.

To improve strength and appearance of the thighs, do exercises 9, 13, 15, 17, 19, 25, 26, 28–30, 35, 42, 44–46, 48, 50, 57–59, 61, 62, 70, 71 and 80–83. You can also do your knee bends with weight bags draped across your shoulders or a barbell resting on them. Climb stairs and mountains whenever you can. After every massage session, do knee bends and exercise 35.

Waist. See Midriff

It is certainly not necessary to do *all* the exercises recommended for any given area every time. It is important to do some daily for any problem you want to correct. It will also be necessary to do every one of these occasionally. You can be almost sure that when you find an exercise that is difficult, you need it. The only answer to that: groan a lot, but do it.

Groups for Exercise

Exercise can be done alone, and it can be done in company. The second way takes more preparation, but is also more fun. If you have friends who, like you, need exercise for whatever reason, invite them over. Use music you all enjoy and have an exercise session. Read over the chapter on vacations and see if there is something you all might want to prepare for. Use the tests, help each other to improve. Co-ed classes are fun and they are challenging. The men aren't going to be outdone by the women, and the women aren't about to give up any ground either. The men will do better with strength exercises and the women with flexibility, but since both types are in this book, the points will be about fifty-fifty. Don't let anybody off the hook either. If Tom doesn't feel like exercising because he got fired, *that's the time he must!* If Evelyn wants to quit because she has discovered she's pregnant, don't hear of it. It's more important then than ever. The only body you have or ever will have is the one you occupy right this minute. If you have let it get out of shape, condition it. If it has been injured, repair it. If it is all that a body should be, keep it that way. What you don't use, you lose. What you use often and well will be all the better for it.

8

Thief of Desire — Stress

"Desire" is a provocative word and denotes an entirely enviable state. If you say to a little boy, "What do you want most in the world?" you will get an immediate, positive, and enthusiastic answer, "A bicycle." His eyes will shine as he describes just the right bicycle, and even if he doesn't get it, just talking about it and hoping for it makes him happy. Ask a thirteen-year-old girl what she most desires and the answer may be, "A horse." Possibly she even knows just the horse, where it is stabled, what his owner wants for him, and exactly how much it will take to transport him and stable him right down the road. As she describes that horse, you may get the impression that thirteen-year-old girls fall in love with horses and you might also think that it was a lucky horse that was so longed for.

When we grow up and leave bicycles and horses behind, we desire love and the special people with whom to share it. Even if, as sometimes happens, we are never able to consummate love with a particular person, it still fills us with joy and contentment just to think about that person, to talk to and about that person, and to hope for occasions just to be in the same room. If, as also often happens, we are able to come close, to be accepted, to love and to be loved, our desires mount higher and higher and our days become merely spaces between nights. But the spaces are filled with sudden rockets of longing, all the more exciting because we can't do anything about them until later. If life is kind, this wondrous condition can continue on and on, and for some it does. For others it doesn't. Why?

There are of course dozens of reasons for the fading of desire that cannot be foreseen and against which we have no protection, but there is a prime reason (maybe *the* reason), which is rarely if ever considered: stress and the unknown capacity of each individual to withstand it.

Stress is characteristic not only of our workdays but also of our relationships with those we're closest to, and that makes us at least in part responsible for those we love. We are also responsible for ourselves and, with the results of studies and experiments now coming in, it becomes more and more evident that we are far more capable of helping ourselves *and others* than our forebears and we have thought.

The field of parapsychology opens a new door every day that reveals lines of communication that are always alive. It is indeed frustrating to realize that most of the time nobody answers the phone when it rings because one or another of the potential communicators is out in the backyard, so to speak, and doesn't hear the bell. There are also lines of communication within ourselves which we are prone to ignore. One of the messages we seem reluctant to recognize is the one our body uses to tell us something about our condition in relation to daily stress and also the more unusual stresses that are hopefully few and far between. Sexual desire is related to stress both directly (you rarely want to make love after losing last year's savings in the market) and indirectly. Of the two, it is the indirect effect that is more damaging, but it is the one you can do most about. Before you can deal intelligently with stress, however, you need some information about it, and about how it affects your body and your desire to make love.

The dictionary starts its description of stress with three words: "pressure," "force," and "strain." Hans Selye, Director of Experimental Medicine and Surgery at the University of Montreal and the man who probably knows the most about stress, claims that each of us enters the world with an inherited capacity to withstand stress. He also says that once this adaptation energy is used up, there is no known way to replace it. So each of us is born with a given capacity to adapt to pressure, force, and strain. But what, exactly, comes under these three headings, and when in life do we start to use up our supply of adaptation energy?

If there are three words that describe birth from a baby's point of view, they would have to be "pressure," "force," and "strain," but he begins at once to add new experiences. The next experience in line would be the stressor known as *change.* You need hardly get your bruised little head past the door to know that the new place is not the same as the one you are leaving, and even if you were to move from here to China you could not experience a more disquieting change than the one you meet on Day One. All the rest of your life, whenever you change addresses, schools, jobs, partners, occupations, and families, your body will have to adapt not only to these changes but also to the chemical changes going on inside the body.

Just as you shoulder your way into this new place, you will receive a blow from a stressor called *discomfort,* as the blazing lights strike your eyes. Your nervous system, as well as your eyes, takes immediate steps to adapt to the painful glare, and all your life your skin will take steps to adapt to the discomfort of cold, heat, and humidity. Your ears will try to protect themselves from destructive noise, your lungs will try to adapt to poisons in the air. Your liver will work overtime to adapt to the foods you eat and whatever you drink. You start to tap your adaptation energy the moment you're born, and you'll use it whenever you're uncomfortable, whether the discomfort is physical or emotional, for the rest of your life.

As you are drawn forth into the world and away from all that was known and safe, you will experience a stressor of singular power, *fear*. Of all the stressors you will meet, fear and anger are the strongest, and they demand the most in adaptation energy. From then on, the assaults on your person come quickly. As you are hung head down for drainage, whacked on the bottom to start your breathing apparatus, cut loose from your mooring, washed, wiped, medicated, and poked, you are meeting another stressor of a high order, *pain*. Your frightened little heart beats wildly, and even then you pour powerful chemicals into your bloodstream to meet the danger. It will be no different in years to come when the dentist begins to drill, the doctor sews up your knee, or you enter the delivery room for a second time. Pain, both acute and chronic, always requires adaptation.

In a matter of a few moments after birth you are taken away from the one thing you know and feel secure with, the mother. It is then that you meet the strongest stressor of all, since it has the power to multiply itself by arousing the stresses of anger, fear and pain too. The name of this prince of stressors is *loss*. When you are finally tucked in your solitary little crib, you will meet the stress of loneliness for the first, not, alas, for the last time.

So when do you start to use up your inherited capacity to withstand stress? At once. How much you will need to expend depends on your life situation, your personality, and, from now on, just how much you know about the price you will have to pay for what you allow to happen. Everything costs, but some things cost more than others, and some are worth far more than others. Getting furious with the garage man because he mangled your clutch may cost exactly the same amount in what might be called "stress points" as three beautiful hours making love. The price is equal, but can you say the same thing for the product?

Your body is possessed of an ancient wisdom. It knows that to survive for your use it must maintain something called *equilibrium*. When you are in this most desirable state of balance, everything feels right.

You are at peace, you feel fine, and your whole body goes about its tasks most cheerfully. When a stress-filled situation occurs or when you are attacked by any one of the many stressors, your body goes into immediate action to put things right and to protect you if necessary. The action is so immediate that you have often made the lifesaving move before you realized it was necessary. Key members in the battery in charge of maintaining *equilibrium* are the adrenals, the two small glands perched above the kidneys. It is the adrenaline poured into your bloodstream by these glands that gives you the sudden strength to lift the Volkswagen off the injured pedestrian or to jump out of harm's way yourself. But these adrenals have another task, and one that is very important—in fact, invaluable—where sex is concerned. They manufacture the male sex hormone, *androgen*, which is responsible for instituting and maintaining erotic desire in both males and females. This hormone is also manufactured in the male testes and in the female ovaries, but if some misadventure should necessitate their removal, sexual desire would continue unabated so long as the adrenals remain intact and functioning. If the adrenals are removed, however, there is a profound drop in sexual interest. And it stands to reason that even when they are not removed, if the adrenals are overworked through too much need to adapt to stress, the price is going to be very high indeed. It is one thing not to make love either by choice or for lack of opportunity, and quite another not to feel anything even approaching sexual desire. Unthinkable! And yet you'd be wise to think about it.

The very best way to keep the adrenals healthy and functioning is to keep the stressors such as anger and fear at bay. To this end it might be well to examine your life for unavoidable stress and for the other kind. If your job drives you up a tree, why not get another? Your wife can't get along without all the advantages your present salary brings her? How do you know? And does she know what the price might eventually be in lonely nights and mounting, unrelieved sexual tension?

Make a list of all the things that make you angry or fill you with anxiety or fear. What things make you feel uptight and who contributes to any of those conditions? What physical things could you change that would bring more equilibrium to your life, and what attitudes could you change in yourself? Getting an upset stomach because the dinner was burned hardly makes sense if you remember that dinners can be replaced but that desire is a far more fragile commodity.

We will always have stress with us, but start now to make choices and decisions. If you will give up the stresses you can manage without, you will be able to hold onto one of the facets of life that you can't do without joyfully—desire.

9

Pain — Preserver of Sexuality

At first glance the title of this chapter is confusing. You are well aware that when you suffered with pleurisy two winters ago, the last thing on your mind was making love. You weren't too interested in it when you broke your leg skiing either, in spite of your proximity to a most attractive, willing, and sympathetic partner. So what, you ask, can pain do for sex other than postpone it? Pain can also postpone aging and maintain youthfulness by helping to protect your self-image as well as your body. It can also enable you to conserve your adaptation energy for the things you want to do in your life, which includes making love. How is this so?

First you have to understand what pain really is besides unpleasant. Pain is an integral part of your closed-circuit-communication system. While your body can handle emergencies without any help from you—emergencies that call for sudden warming or cooling, a step-up in oxygen supply, sudden processing of food to increase your fuel supply and the simultaneous closing down of systems such as digestion and excretion—there are some things that make your assistance imperative. Pain will scream at you to get your hand off the hot stove, and its jangling tocsin will make it impossible to walk on a smashed ankle. Pain will inform you of secret decay in a tooth and give the signal when it is time to start for the hospital's delivery room. Those are orders you will not be able to ignore. It's the pain you *can* ignore that we need to look into.

Pain is not merely an unpleasant by-product of living; it has a job to do, and it always means something.

Each of us reacts to pain according to the examples we have been set in our early years, our personalities, and our pain thresholds. What might be terribly upsetting, even agonizing, for one person may merely nag another. While a high pain threshold is helpful in conserving one's adaptation energy, it is less helpful in another way. Unless pain really shakes us up, many of us tend to ignore it and we think we are being strong. At first we "grin and bear it," and later, when the condition has settled in and become chronic, we substitute the "try to live with it" attitude. Both attitudes are wrong, shortsighted, and very destructive; they should be labeled POISON.

The poison ingested through putting up with pain attacks on many fronts and the one most closely connected with our happiness is the area called the subconscious. The subconscious has the eye of an eagle and misses nothing we do, nor the way in which we do it. It has the ear of an Indian and can tap in on every conversation we have and is especially attentive to those we hold with ourselves. It forgets nothing and never sleeps. To see the results of such constant awareness, look hard and long at every old person you see. Their bodies are the culmination of all they have done, suffered, and thought about. Their bodies may also tell you that they neglected to lavish even a fraction of the care they gave their houses and conveyances on their bodies.

Many old people are bent and many limp noticeably. Most take short steps and move awkwardly. Almost all sit down very slowly and carefully, sometimes letting go and falling the last inch or so. They rise in sections, often with audible sounds of lesser or greater distress. They cannot run, and many are unable to pick up their pace at all, which may account for their high mortality rate as pedestrians—that and the fact that their necks and shoulders are often so stiff and painful that they can't easily look up and down the highway before crossing. Failing muscle control and a lack of balance cause some old people to fall when taking a sudden step to the back or side, and this accounts for their high incidence of hip injuries. All problems which progress to that extreme do so through default. These folks stopped using their necks, shoulders, backs, legs, and feet for a variety of reasons—most of which could have been corrected and wiped off the slate through proper care, leaving them in a position to enjoy the years of wisdom and, for many, total freedom from toil.

You begin to age the day you are born, and what you are like at the far end of life depends on what you do in the beginning and on what you continue with, day by day from then on. The built-in protection that warns you when anything is amiss is pain. The end result will be due in large part to the way you handle pain and whether or not you understand its messages. Old people who have fallen into disrepair are suffering from conditions that have become chronic, either with actual chronic pain or the fear of remembered pain. The fear of remembered pain lies deep in the subconscious, and it has a way of limiting motion even when the cause has been removed. The habit of protecting painful parts of ourselves lingers on, causing the very limitation of movement we try to prevent through corrective exercises. It is these limiting, protective movements that cause the appearance of being old, even at age forty. It is freedom from such limitation, plus enjoyment of life, that gives a youthful appearance even at sixty.

Unattended pain can do a bang-up job on your self-image. Let's take a very common example. You begin to have headaches whenever you have a lot of reading to do, but because you have a lot of reading to do as well as many other chores, you treat the symptom, pain, rather than investigate the cause. Depending on what your parents or partners do for headaches, you may take a couple of aspirin (there's no such thing as one), lie down in a darkened room, drink some herb tea, or you may square your shoulders and get on with the job. The pain may go away temporarily or it may just damp down to a dull throb, but you will continue to strain your eyes, which are doing their best to adapt to a condition of disequilibrium. There goes some of your limited supply of adaptation energy, but that isn't all that happens by any means. The small muscles around your eyes are constantly being tightened to narrow your field of vision and bring what you see into sharper focus. These are joined by the muscles between your eyes and the many neighboring muscles in face and forehead. These are the same muscles that react to pain with tension. You can locate them simply by squinting and thinking how you'd feel if you were in considerable pain. Then look in the mirror; the mask you see there sets a little tighter every time you either grimace with pain or squint to see. Lines thus caused are lines of strain, not of laughter, and soon that face in the mirror will look tired, strained, and unhappy. When you see that reflection, you think, "My God! I look terrible, I need some rest." (Actually you need glasses.) And your subconscious sees that face too. It registers *I look terrible,* and that message, without any modifications attached, goes right into your computer. Continue this way over many months and you will have ample opportunity to repeat that message over and over, with predictable reinforcement. Repetition amounts to amplification. That's what makes a chance remark from another person carry so much weight. "Darling, you look so tired," comes very close to "I look terrible." Sometimes we even move the words around and hear, "Darling, you look terrible," because that's what we expect to hear. Headaches mean something, and pain is one guardian angel that can cut through your preoccupation, if you will let it.

Then there is emotional pain, and almost nobody escapes without experiencing it. Let's say you have blundered into a job that just isn't for you. However, the pay is good, the hours are okay, and one of these days when the bills let up, you'll look around for something else. But "one of these days" runs into years (it may take only months), and you become so uptight that you have to work harder and harder to accomplish less and less. Several minor symptoms begin to plague you. Your digestion is disturbed and you take an antacid, your head aches and you take aspirin. You develop insomnia and begin taking sleeping pills; you feel exhausted, even in the morning, so you take Dexedrine, which makes you feel nervous, and so you take Valium. You bark at your family, your secretary, and your father, who asked if anything is bothering you. But you don't see the warning signals until something finally gives way, usually the weakest link in your body chain and also the site you have chosen as a target for your tension. Even then you don't tie effect to cause. It usually happens like this.

The attention-getting episode rarely happens at the office or wherever the trouble lies, but somewhere else after some additional stress overloads the circuit. Let's say you have just spent a very unpleasant weekend with some relatives. On the way home you feel some tightness in your lower back, which becomes increasingly painful the nearer you get to home. When you finally arrive and step out of your car, you can't straighten up. You hobble into the house, lower yourself into your chair very carefully, and call for aspirin and a martini. You feel a little better after dinner and attribute your trouble to the long drive, a cold draft, the heavy suitcases. Anything will do. The pain gigs you again when you get out of your chair, and you spend a sleepless night trying to find a comfortable position. The next morning it is still with you, and so is the feeling that one wrong move will immobilize you in an agonizing bent-over position. You come down the stairs sideways, holding onto the banister. Have you seen old people do that? Well, this is the way it starts. You'd feel justified staying at home, but the board is meeting to consider a proposal put forth by your department, and you must be there. You manage somehow, and when two members express strong opposition to your views, you are not only disappointed but frustrated as well. They are the two members who always upset plans, and they are also the two who know nothing much about the business. You would like to knock their heads together. At lunch you are offered your favorite table with its seat against the wall, but you have to ask the headwaiter for a different one with a straight-backed chair. Not only have you been denied the expected triumph at the office, but you feel grumpy, defeated, and old. On the drive home the traffic seems worse than usual, and getting out of the car is even harder than the night before. There isn't a chance in the world of keeping your badminton date, but you send your wife along without you. The show on TV is a bore, but you hurt too much to get up and change it. You elect to stay home the next day and the next, and by the following weekend you are no better. That means no tennis and no golf either. Sunday is your anniversary, and you spend the evening lying on an electric heating pad.

What you have just suffered is called an "acute episode," and about half the population suffers one of these at least once in a lifetime; many, especially ex-athletes, suffer many more. That is not because of their active youths, but because active youths (and their female counterparts) often sustain muscle tears in sports —tears which heal almost at once, especially if one continues to be active, but which leave what are called "trigger points" at the site of the injury. These trigger points are not heard from again unless tension has taken up residence in that area. Typical of such spots are the lower back muscles, the gluteals, and the chest and shoulder muscles. Then the trigger point goes into spasm, bringing as many neighboring muscles along as possible. They even cause what is called referred pain, far from the site of the original injury; a good example is the pain radiating down the leg from a "point" deep in the buttocks.

The usual method used in treating the kind of acute back pain that has no apparent pathology—such as "arthritis" or a "disc"—is bedrest, aspirin, moist heat, an analgesic ointment, and antispasm medication, plus the advice to "take it easy for a while." Taking it easy is usually interpreted to mean "Don't play tennis, don't play golf, don't lift anything heavy, and get lots of rest." Since few people use exercises as protective devices (those who do almost never have back pain), nobody ever mentions it in connection with post-episode recuperation. So the tension sets in harder, and even when the pain is either gone entirely or is so minimal you feel you can "live with it," you don't do the one thing that will help—move. Rest and medication won't chase your tension away, especially when you dose yourself with tension liberally and daily at the office, and so you become a "back cripple"—someone who either has back pain or lives in fear of having another painful episode. You give up the sports you enjoyed and you avoid driving too long, standing too long, and sitting too long. You put on weight, you feel sluggish and depressed. Your wife has been reading *The Joy of Sex* and just left it on your night table; you suspect she is trying to tell you something. She is.

Your pain has been trying to tell you something too, for almost a year. It has been trying to get you to pay some attention to the *cause* of your trouble rather than the symptoms. You are tense and uptight. You are under far more pressure than you can equalize with the physical outlets at your disposal. Even the exercise you enjoyed before the back spasms began wasn't enough for that kind of tension. Your pain has been warning you day after painful day that you are using up your adaptation energy hand over fist, as though there were no tomorrow. Your self-image is taking a terrible beating as you turn down invitations to join your friends on the court and your wife on her side of the bed. If, when the trouble had first started, you had said to yourself, "What's a young fellow like you doing with a creaky back?" and if you had known that backaches are very rare without the company of their running mate, tension, you might have faced the problem: your job. You've been telling yourself for too long that it is only temporary; now your back is telling you that whatever the advantages of the status quo, the price is too high. The time for change is *almost* at hand.

Before you can do anything drastic, you will need to regain your faith in your physical self and get rid of the exhaustion that gets out of bed with you each morning. You will have to get rid of your backache. For the short and immediate haul, you will need the *limbering series* on pages 64–72. You will need to do them every few hours all day long until the underlying, warning tightness has disappeared. If your doctor will give you a prescription for a coolant spray, use it *and the exercises* at the first twinge, as well as at stipulated times—upon rising, midmorning, before lunch, midafternoon, on arriving home, midevening, and before bed.

As soon as you have regained control of your body and its pain, you will need to get involved in some very active sports. To get rid of the day's accumulated tension you could jog a couple of miles each evening. If any morning is particularly rough, skip lunch and go to the club or the Y and swim laps. And then get out of that job. However, you won't be able to face this change until you feel well. Constant pain and exhaustion will work against self-confidence, as does the anxiety that always accompanies chronic pain and disability. So, unless you do something about your back, you won't be capable of changing the working situation that caused your back problem in the first place. And don't stop with merely healing your back, for if you do nothing about the underlying situation, you may simply move the site of your tension target from your back to a very different area. It is quite possible to develop ulcers, colitis, or a nervous breakdown. It is equally possible and, according to statistics, all too probable that you may, with the help of unremitting stress and the constant outpouring of stress hormones, get your heart to try for the big one. That would change your situation drastically indeed, and you wouldn't have to be involved in the decision at all.

Unattended pain is the great ager. Look again at old people and notice how *bound* they seem to be. They really are bound. Can you remember how you felt the last time you had the flu? Your neck hurt and your back ached. Your legs were stiff and painful, and so were your shoulders. You felt miserable. Well, that's how chronic pain feels, and it doesn't go away when your fever drops back to normal. All chronic pain was once acute, and pain that is acute is signaling *new* trouble. Trouble that is new is the kind with the best chance of correction, but all too often it is ignored until the original problem has increased to the point where it can no longer be pushed into the background and you finally seek help. "When did you first notice the pain?" often elicits the answer, "Well, Doc, I really don't remember. I sure had it when I was shoveling snow last winter, but then I remember some difficulty when we raked up the yard last fall. . . . Wait a minute, I had it last spring too, and my wife had to put in the garden."

The *bound* look of the old comes when the painful condition is allowed to become chronic and the effort to avoid the pain causes the sufferer to hold certain muscles rigid over long periods of time. This shortens the muscles and robs them of their resiliency; the shortening then affects the joints and bones, pulling them out of line, and the body out of balance. This can happen so slowly as to go unnoticed for a long time. The limp you walk with when an old knee or hip injury flares may become a habit and continue after the acute episode is a thing of the past; this is especially true when daily work enforces limitation of movement. Deep in the subconscious there is the programmed information that a shortened step prevents sudden twinges of pain in that knee or hip. Then the shortened step shortens the muscles further, and that causes discomfort—not enough to make you ask yourself, "What's a young fellow like me doing with a bum knee or hip?" but just enough to make you walk a little more carefully than a young fellow should have to walk. Not enough to make you wonder why you have a bad back, just enough to cause you to be careful getting into and out of chairs. Not enough to make you curious about your shoulder when your tennis serve lacks power and you subconsciously put a brake on your swing. Not enough to make you give up skiing, but quite enough to make you unwittingly favor your football knee by making as many turns to the right as the slope will allow so that the uninjured left leg can take the brunt of the action.

To keep your body fit for life, for love and loving, you need to be constantly aware of what is going on in your body. You also need to develop a very high level of expectation. You should *expect* to be comfortable and free from pain. You should *expect* your muscles to perform with well-oiled efficiency. You should *expect* complete recovery if you are injured, have a baby, or fall ill. Don't settle for anything less, and never agree to "try to live with it." It would be far better to make every possible effort to keep yourself in top running order.

Check out any creaky joints, shortened muscles, or posture anomalies that could lead to imbalance and force you to use vital adaptation energy needlessly . . . and check your life. You won't be afraid to change it if your health is fine and your body strong. *One keypoint: never ignore a physical or an emotional pain. To do so is to rob it of its assigned work as a warner and spotter of trouble and to make it an agent in the service of early aging, and an enemy of health and happiness.*

10

How Do Your Signals Read?

Back in the fifties when we were giving the test for minimum muscular fitness to thousands of schoolchildren, we reaped a bonus harvest. Not only did we learn about their muscular fitness or the lack of it, we learned about masks and how to see behind them. All of us wear masks some of the time, and there are people who never take them off, even when they are alone. Behind our masks we hide our hurts, our anxieties, fears, irritations, and angers. We also hide our longings and our loneliness and to the extent that our masks are successful shields, we are also misunderstood.

The very young children who came to us to be tested (except those who had been emotionally damaged) wore no masks. As they approached our tables we could see curiosity, friendliness, anxiety, or any of several degrees of fear. Probably because they kept coming at us—class after class of six-, seven-, and eight-year-olds, thousands of them—without any let-up for weeks on end, we began to notice the many signals they displayed with their bodies. The ones who had fear in their faces either said nothing at all or talked too much. (Have you ever noticed how you chatter to your dentist?) The fearful children also folded their arms across their chests and bunched up their shoulders. The ones who were not troubled at all about the new experience either said a casual hello to our greetings or just grinned as they hopped up onto the table. Their arms hung free and their shoulders were completely relaxed. When they were told to lie down for the first test, the very fearful simply couldn't do it. They were terrified of laying their bodies open to attack. Often it took gentle persuasion and helping hands before they would chance it. Many could not let their arms fall back on the table when their hands were clasped behind their necks, but hugged their ears protectively with their bent arms. Another similar sign coming from fearful children was holding one knee bent over the other and their bodies turned slightly away from the tester once they were fully supine. One glance at their faces and you knew you were seeing not only fear, but a kind of hopeless desperation. Later, when the test was over and they were told they could get down, many of them were more concerned about keeping their legs tightly pressed together than with negotiating the descent safely. While we didn't give the crotch test (page 33) at that time, we have since added it to our battery and we have found that these fearful children have already shortened the muscles of their inner thighs. Most of the fearful ones, when they said anything at all, would whisper "I can't" when asked to sit up for the first test. And often it was quite true, they couldn't. They were generally weak and had inflexible backs and hamstrings (Test 6), and they were the ones who often failed two or more tests. This was unheard of in Europe, but 22 percent of our children were in this category. When teachers were asked about the children with multiple failures they referred to them as "characters" or "troubled youngsters."

When we moved into the junior high school we saw at once that there was a difference: those children all seemed to have the same expression. There was a kind of blankness in their eyes that every teacher will recognize. It is not a sign of absence, but rather one of caution. There was much less chatter and almost all of them, even the confident children, were watchful and quiet. But other things did not change at all. The fearful approached the tables with their arms hugging their chests, or shoulders pulled up and pressed forward. They didn't say they couldn't lie down but they often raised one knee slightly and covered the other as they turned a little away. Their elbows rarely lay flat and open on the table. They didn't say they couldn't sit up in tests 1 and 2, but before trying, many gave excuses for expected poor performance with "I fell in gym and I'm not sure I can." They too got off the table as though their ankles were tied together. Those with multiple failures were still designated as "characters" by their teachers.

At the high-school level the masks were firmly in place, but now certain vocal signals were being sounded. "Yah! It's a pipe!" or "What did you say this test was for?" or occasionally, "I hurt my back last week . . . I don't know if . . ." The self-assured were still relaxed and took the test with ease, getting down from the tables using first one leg and then the other in a single fluid motion. The anxious and the fearful approached as usual, with chest-shielding arms and strained shoulders, but now there was a difference. Their postures were set. It wasn't this new experience which caused tension and an immediate but temporary posture change. Now there was no other way to stand even in very relaxed situations. They were now prisoners of habit begun many years before when perhaps there had been reason to fear. The sad thing was that these signals triggered certain reactions in people who saw them. The confident, open youngster is always accepted quicker and more fully than one who appears to slink furtively, and who looks both secretive and somehow afraid. There is always less resistance to the easy, welcoming sort of person while an almost palpable social barrier is presented to the person who can handle it least. Unhappily, having created the resistance in others through body signals, the poor sender (who is often all too sensitive when it comes to receiving signals) senses the resistance in the others. Then he nods to himself, saying, "See, they just don't like me." And sure enough, they don't, but not one could give you a good sound reason. It usually boils down to "It's just a feeling."

Your body sends out signals all the time. No matter what your words say, your body will give you away to anyone with the wit or sensitivity to read you. If people are sensitive, whether they've made a study of body signals or not, they will read you subconsciously and react accordingly, sometimes with equally inappropriate behavior. However, if they do understand at least something about body signals (both their own and those of others) and are interested in people as those in love are interested in each other, then they can observe with understanding and react in such a way as to open the shells of the lonely, remove the stings from the hostile, and even draw close to those who for some reason—usually beyond both knowledge or control—are afraid of love, afraid to love, and afraid to be loved.

It would be very helpful to know something about the body signals we all use, and read and react to subconsciously. We could then put them to conscious use, both in reading others and in *consciously* affecting their subconscious reactions to us. There is something else of value. If, at the height of an angry exchange, we should suddenly catch ourselves signaling anger through body attitude or movement, while at the same time we are *saying* that there is no reason whatever for this altercation, we confuse, frustrate and worsen the situation. Anger is a stressor, and when one's days are spattered with such exchanges, it is almost impossible to bring the full force of sexual desire to bear at night.

While everyone's emotional mannerisms are slightly different, the direction they take have a surprising similarity. If we are talking and I turn my back on you, there is little doubt that I don't wish to see your point. I can do the same thing a little less obviously by turning my head and looking out of the window or by doodling. If I want to tell you that I am interested in you and I look long and earnestly into your face, you can't miss it.

However, I might not want to show you everything I feel for you just in case you are not the slightest bit interested. I could easily condense that look into a quick, intense one and run no risk at all of rejection. The only risk would be that you would miss it. So if you are interested in someone, keep your eyes open.

If I were furious with you I might want to do what I did without the slightest compunction when I was eight years old—let you have one on the nose. As an adult I no longer express myself so directly, but if you look at my fists (in or out of my pockets) you can read me right down to the white knuckles. You know what's in my mind even when my words say something quite different. You can then make a choice, but first make a quick check on your own fists. Are they also balled? If so, you must know that my subconscious is reading you quite well and our combined angers are reinforcing each other. Your choices are to stay or to leave, but if you stay and continue to shout (even silently), we'll get nowhere. However, if you relax your shoulders, open your hands, and put them where I can see them, my subconscious may take note and back down too. Your other choice, to leave, needs handling too. Turning on your heel and walking out will only prolong the time of stress. My eight-year-old self would have thrown a block at the back of your frustrating head. Angry adults bear a striking resemblance to angry eight-year-olds. Make some reasonable excuse and promise to return to the "discussion." When you do come back, watch carefully for the signals which will tell you what my mood and attitude really are. They may have flipped sunny-side-up. If you look carefully at me, you tell me you are interested. If you sit down easily with relaxed and open hands in full sight, you could take the anger right out of me and not have to say anything more than, "Sorry I took so long." If I am still sitting with protective and defensive arms folded over my chest and crossed legs—which all but shout, "To the battlements!"—it would be best to find a reason to put off the encounter. The first time you pass my door and see me leaning back in my chair, relaxed and open, try again.

Sometimes we are tempted to say to our loved ones, "I never know whether you really want to go or not." Watch their bodies when you propose the trip and you can tell. The person filled with enthusiasm twists in his chair and may slide forward, as if all set to start for the door even if the occasion won't arrive till next June. If your idea is met with a sudden crossing of legs or arms, there's resistance. No signal taken by itself is conclusive, of course, but they are all straws in the wind. If I say, "Yup, that's a great idea," and I don't slide forward in my chair, cock my head a little, look you straight in the eye, but I do cross my legs or fold my arms over my chest and perhaps even turn a little away from you, then you know that it would be better to try something else. Oh, I'll go of course, because I know you want to; but my body will be signaling boredom and you won't have much fun . . . and I won't even know that's what I'm telling you.

It is always a mistake to put another person on the spot. Always. We all have faults, we all err from time to time. For most of us the knowledge that we aren't perfect is rather hard to take. We feel even more uncomfortable when others know it. Discomfort of any sort is a stressor and uses up adaptation energy uselessly, energy that may be needed for combating disease, falling in love, or just getting through the day twenty years from now. You may be entirely right in your accusations, you may have caught someone dead center, red-handed, and in the cookie jar, but if you make an issue of it right then, you may well win your point and lose your friend. The fly on the end of your pin will hide his hands, fold his arms, cross his legs, and look away. Nothing is gained except an enemy.

Of course, you can blunder into something by accident. The other person is usually aware of your proximity to thin ice long before you are, and may clasp hands while rubbing thumbs together, pick cuticle, or even bite nails. If you are wise, when you see these signals you will backtrack. It is far better to learn something in good time than to roar in with guns ablaze or fall into the treacle headfirst.

Lovers rarely hurt each other in this way, but irate parents often forget that forbearance, patience, and understanding are properties of love. They do not realize that *they* set the patterns and attitudes that will either bear their children up through the years or drag them down, often to utter misery. Almost no parent gives any thought to the expenditure of adaptation energy when it comes to children. But a child can live under such stress in a house so filled with anger that there is little left when he reaches the freedom that adulthood might bring. If your loved one has the telltale shape of bitten nails from childhood, you might wonder whether certain defensive habits and attitudes which seem totally inappropriate were not instituted long ago by an angry, insensitive putter-downer. People who have never been used in this way are rarely defensive, but the one who suffered often and deeply is defensive forever. The cure lies in forgetting, but one cannot forget past miseries when a reasonable facsimile keeps recurring. One of the loveliest things about falling in love is the first blooming of absolute trust. When that trust exists you share everything, all the joys of the present and all the sorrows of the past. If you will but listen carefully to all the sorrows and all the hurts that are described to you, and if you will act upon that information by never recreating them in any way, you will bind your love to you with unbreakable bonds. The wounds that are laid on us as adults can be evaluated and discarded. The ones that wounded us as helpless children are there for the duration. They are like barely contained fires which need only the slightest breeze to blaze into a major conflagration. If you know and understand what hurt your love as a child, you will never reduce that person to angry helplessness as an adult.

Possession is a funny thing. If people feel that something (or someone) is totally theirs, they rarely need to show it. If they are not quite certain, then it becomes imperative that they give signals of ownership. If you watch two people who are deeply in love but who aren't in a position to show it, you see two people who don't need to come close, even to touch fingers; just knowing the other is near suffices. When people are not that sure of possession, then a great deal of touching, patting shoulders, straightening of clothing, even grooming, will be bestowed by the uncertain partner. These are all signals that others are supposed to see. This bit of information is useful to both the touched and the toucher, especially if the person on the receiving end of the touching loves the toucher and wants to give happiness and, in this instance, reassurance.

The age of fourteen is a time when kids watch everything adults do, partly because it's a habit and partly because they'd rather do things in an acceptable manner than be embarrassed by making faux pas. I remember when I was that age that I once noticed two old marrieds sitting at a table in a restaurant. During the entire meal neither of them said one single word to the other. They looked so cold, so locked in, and so *lonely* that I swore right then and there that such a calamity would never overtake me—but it did. We become so used to each other that we forget to watch, and when we don't watch we miss all the things that are said, even in silence. Among the many nonverbal signs of anger and frustration are slammed doors and drawers, heavy footsteps, rattled dishes, and kicked walls. Sorrow and despair elicit long, deep-drawn breaths—not from everyone and not all the time, but if you hear them, worry. Why is the other sad? Did you cause it? Can you help? There are signs of loving and acceptance too. You may say nothing at all during the meal, but one may lay a hand over the other's, touch a cheek, pass something that was not requested. Such gestures say that things are just fine. "Be silent if you will, I am here and we are together."

Touching is a very important line of communication

and it carries unmistakable messages. The hand that scratches behind a dog's ear conveys all the affection the dog craves. The hand laid gently on a child's head is far more eloquent than whole pages of praise. The often absentminded caresses of lovers touch even the hearts of onlookers. Last spring I was having lunch with some friends in an outdoor restaurant. There was a fountain at the other end of the lawn and two young people watching as the spray mixed with the sunlight in a cascade of rainbows. The girl's arm was around the boy's waist and his hand patted and caressed her hip the way one might smooth the back of a silken cat. He was totally unaware of what he was doing, but it wasn't long before every diner was. Far from causing critical smirks, as the eyes of the various people met, understanding seemed to follow and they would smile. Most of the people there were of an older generation to whom such license had never been permitted and yet each read the message of love and affection in the gesture. The looks they silently exchanged at each table seemed to say, "Nice to see young folks in love."

Whom do you touch and how do you touch them? The surest way to cement love that is at its tenuous beginning is to touch. The surest way to undermine love and self-confidence is never to touch someone who needs to be touched. Years ago there was a ruling in the public schools that no teacher might ever touch a child. This might have been an extreme interpretation of the rule that no teacher could smack a child, but there it stood. In my exercise school, where hundreds came each week to be taught exercise and tumbling, the rule was to touch and touch often. The teachers were shown how to put a hand on a small shoulder so that the thumb rested on the collarbone and the fingers reached toward the spine. The warm, affectionate hand was like a blanket draped over the shoulder. No reaching or grasping, no overwhelming hugs, just a gentle pressure that said, "Friend." At the close of each class the teacher shook hands with each little person and said "O.K.,

Johnny," and added some little message about how he had done and then asked "What color are my eyes?" That meant that every child was spoken to by name, told something about himself or herself, and then each had to make eye contact with heads up and backs straight. "They're blue, Eleanor . . . and thank you." All the while, the hand was held in a firm, warm grip.

Our teachers were not selected for proficiency at gymnastics; that came second. They were chosen for their ability to pour forth warmth, love, and encouragement. When it was time for a tumbling lesson, none of those teachers said, "Go and practice." It was always, "Come and try and I will catch you." Gentle, safe, sure hands turned little people upside down and over. They patterned little bodies to move surely and with beauty and rhythm; they caught handstands, directed walkovers and cartwheels, and everywhere there was praise, kindness, and understanding. The place was alive with it. It was because of this feeling conveyed through praise, tone of voice, and *touch* that youngsters came back year after year until they went away to college. It is what they look for now for their children.

Everyone has a reservoir of warmth and love. The trick in tapping it is in the development of self-confidence. People whose experience with being accepted, liked, and loved has been constant from babyhood, have that self-confidence. They know others like them and want to be with them. With that knowledge they are completely free from any fear of rejection. Their open faces and easy relaxed bodies not only invite encounter, they make it seem both natural and desirable, even to people who usually find opening up to others very difficult. The person lacking in such self-confidence might be a very warm soul, longing to come close to others, but his fear of rejection is so strong that he can't open the door to welcome someone in. He cannot even find a way to let himself out.

It is possible, by means of studied movements, to send warm and welcoming messages to others, and it is possible through the use of these same movements to instruct ourselves. Actors and actresses do it all the time. They have only to know what mood is expected for the part to provide it. So can you. If you feel unsure as you enter a room filled with people and you have a tendency to slide around the door with head down and shoulders rounded, make a note of it and change it. If you would like to be more open and acceptable to people but find your arms closing around yourself every time you are on display, even at a PTA meeting or standing with a group in ordinary conversation, make a note of that. If you find that your fellow workers don't take to you even though you want very much to be accepted, ask yourself what sort of signals you are sending. Watch yourself and watch others, the ones you would like to know. How do they move, stand, hold their arms? Compare their mannerisms with yours. The exercises in this book can free you of old habits and leave you prepared for change if you will make the effort to note what needs changing. Even if you aren't sure at first, there is something you can work on right away—tension. Tension signals are the easiest to spot and hardest to control. When people are tense they give off a feeling of uneasiness, and others tend to be warded off. Tension mounts in people for a variety of reasons, but there is no reason to accept its limitations. The quickest way to release tension and thereby allow your body and mind to relax is through physical activity. Physical activity also helps build the drive needed by the lethargic personality. Check with all the tests and problems, locate your deficiencies, and set up a program designed to change them. Watch both the signals you send and those sent by others. Life does not change by itself; outside influences change it or we change it. Outside influences are unpredictable and could make things worse, so take the initiative yourself. Decide what you want changed and do it yourself.

People who are sexually aware of themselves move differently from those who are not. Sometimes the tension they put into their walk and the way they stand and sit is conscious, but most of the time it is totally unconscious. The reception of those signals is also unconscious. Eyes may register that the other person is attractive, or doing well out there on the court, or is certainly a good dancer, or perhaps should stick to rock and leave the fox trot alone. But the underlying sexuality being noted is coming in through another receiver. Unless you know what to look for, the subtle forward thrust of the pelvis and the tightening of the buttocks muscles will be missed. A woman with a low level of sexuality who wants to portray a sexy walk can swing her hips from one side of the road to the other and no heads will be turned among passing pedestrians. The healthy, sexually aware woman scarcely has to move at all. In fact, she can stand perfectly still and yet manage to convey her confidence and sexuality to both men and women the second they lay eyes on her. And, naturally, a man can and does convey the same message. The reception of this condition is not uniform, however, and depends entirely on the receiver. If the receiver has a hang-up about sex, he or she may take an instant dislike to the individual without having the slightest idea why. If there is a chance that comparisons will be made and that the receiver will come off second best, the same unearned dislike may be generated. However, if the receiver is in what is called "courtship readiness," there may be instant recognition and attraction. Whatever the reception, the sexually aware person will go right on displaying. There is virtually no way to turn it off, but how do you turn it on?

Pelvis Power

Several years before Elvis popularized the pelvis, I had been asked to conduct preseason ski classes by a ski club of about fifty couples. It was a new club and most of them were fairly new to skiing. Now, a person with normal muscle condition, a sense of rhythm, the ability to tilt the pelvis under (exercises 38, 41, 42, 44, and 45), and about four hours of exercises using basic skiing form, can learn to ski well enough in a gym to go down a gentle slope, turn right and left and stop, the first hour he gets out on the hill. By afternoon this same neophyte can ski much steeper pitches with everything under control.

Since the gym was not very large and we would be using skis as well as exercises, we split the class: fifty women in the morning session and their fifty husbands at night. In skiing as in so many sports, the ability to direct the positioning of the pelvis is absolutely essential. If you can't tuck your pelvis under, you cannot get your weight forward onto the front of the skis, and it is then impossible to control their direction. A fall is inevitable. That first morning I began to teach the weight-forward position with the standing pelvic tilt (exercise 44). The ladies were standing in a circle with feet apart, knees bent, and their hands resting on their thighs close to their bent knees. I said, "Push your seats out and arch your backs. Pretend you are little kids and you are watching a caterpillar on the floor in front of you. Now, someone comes along with a canoe paddle and swats your seat. The rules say you can't run away, you can't stand straight or let go of your knees. Where would your seats go?" I expected to see every pelvis in the room tuck under and the seats disappear. *Not one did.* I was surprised. If you consider that a pelvic tilt for skiing and a pelvic tilt for making love are identical, why couldn't women who obviously were in a position to use it for the latter activity tilt? My next thought was that they must have very strong, active, and slender husbands. If you can burn up twenty calories a minute when you share equally in the "work," think how much you'd burn up if all the work fell to one partner! That night I got the shock of my life: only five out of that group of fifty husbands could tilt worth a darn. I wondered vaguely what who did to whom and how they made out with it.

I decided to teach more than skiing to that group, but I knew better than to say what I was planning to teach. I explained in very technical language why the weight had to be forward and how they were to get it there, and using every exercise you have in this book in the section on the pelvis, I worked them mercilessly. By the end of the week some of them were fantastic, a few were suspicious, but all of them could tilt. By the time there was snow on the slopes they could also ski, but it was two years before I learned that my technical language had fooled almost no one. By the end of the second lesson most of them had caught on, but while my ruse hadn't worked in one way (they knew what I was up to) it had in another; it allowed them to do what they wanted to do and what they knew they ought to do, but were too inhibited to do except under the guise of ski exercises. That was when I started my crusade for better lovemaking. That was when I wrote the chapter on "Sexercise" and put it in a book. That was when every member of my school, from three-year-olds up, started to learn the pelvic tilt . . . and they were excellent students. Not once did anyone question me on the purpose of the exercises. That was because I beat them to the punch. For girls it was the best exercise for sitting to a canter on a horse, for boys it was essential when a bat was swung, and for everyone it was a ski exercise. They believed me because it happened to be the truth.

Within a short time, I began to notice that the men and women in my classes who were using the tilt so often and so well began to walk differently, stand differently, and even sit differently. I couldn't say what it was at first, it was just *there*. Later I realized that these people now felt something to be different *in* their bodies. This then affected the way they thought *about* their bodies. It wasn't too much later that it began to be a joke in our town that I seemed to be running a marriage bureau. The sexual awareness was not only affecting the people who were developing it, but was getting through to others. They began noticing each other, and not just with their eyes, which are usually prejudiced in favor of obvious good looks. They began to sense warmth, subtle attraction, and sexual tension. What a lovely way to even out the inequality that starts when heredity presents you with features you wish had stayed on your mother's side of the family.

The following summer I had a chance to use this discovery in a concentrated way, not for people just entering the courtship stage, but for those who were quite settled in their marriages or who were ready to start another. I had set up a ten-day fitness camp at a YMCA facility and twenty-eight women applied. They ranged in age from nineteen to sixty, most were interested in losing weight, one wanted to gain, and three just wanted to get into better condition.

We started with the tests the first morning and they revealed a great deal of inflexibility, caused for the most part by tension, which is not dissipated through physical activity, but stored instead. Crotch flexibility was poor for many, which indicated considerable inhibition—not unusual in those days. Girls who swung their hips weren't considered "nice," and above all things it was important to be thought of as "nice," whatever that meant. I knew I had to get those hips swinging and the pelvises tilting, and all I had was ten days. Ten days versus years for some, and a lifetime for others. Shock treatment was indicated, but what would shock "gently raised" ladies that they would still accept as necessary? I had had a sauna put in for the course and there was a beautiful outdoor swimming pool. I don't know when I had begun to understand the part played in sexuality by nature, but I did know it was powerful and I decided to give it a chance. Available were sun, air, water, a forest, and a flowering field.

Each morning we began the day with a walk through the silent forest, silent except for our footsteps and low voices. I knew by the soft tones that the magic had begun. Next we worked on the exercise floor all morning, to wild and wonderful music, every bit of which had a tantalizing and sexy beat. They were tired by noon, but it was a nice, loose, relaxed tired which would be gone after an hour of rest. I suggested they take their blankets into the field and get a tan. Most of them went. That afternoon we used the same music and I had them working outdoors in the hot sun. They had been in the pool twice that day, once in the morning and once after the exercise class in the afternoon. They thought that would end the day. Not a bit of it. We had some talk on the deck after dinner and then they were told to get on down to the sauna at nine. All were to be ready to sweat—as if they hadn't all day.

When I joined the group in the sauna, they looked like a convention of mummies all wrapped up in sheets and towels. I have found that asking children or anyone else if they want to do something is a mistake, so I said to the first ten near the door, "Off with the sheets and into the sauna." They obediently left their sheets behind and filed in. When they came out and grabbed for the sheets again I said, "Now, while you are all hot and steaming, head for the pool. It's the extreme changes in temperature that will exercise your pores to open and close—that's what you are after." It may or may not have been true, but it gave them something to think about, and off they went. The next group dropped their sheets and went into the sauna. They didn't need to be told to go to the pool either, they went along on their own—and very happily.

The next day they seemed far more relaxed, especially through the shoulders. They were also more able and willing to swing and tilt. The second night one of my assistants took over, and there wasn't a dissenting murmur as the evening's activities began. By the third night, there was no longer any sheet grabbing and I had told them that since their sunbathing area in the field was completely private they should feel free to get all-over tans if they wanted. Many did. There was, however, one standout.

One lady had managed to avoid the sauna and evening dip altogether. She said she minded the heat, which is quite legitimate; not everyone can take it. But I had noticed that she was a good swimmer and went in twice each day. I sought her out on the third night and said, "Come on, it's time you joined the others in the pool." She replied, "I just can't, I'm too embarrassed. All my life I've been told what an ugly body I had and that I should keep it covered." She didn't have an ugly body at all, but someone had certainly done a job on her self-image. I told her it wasn't true but that, if she felt embarrassed, I could understand it and I had a plan. "You can wear your suit into the water and then take it off for your swim. Then you can put it back on. No one will see you and you can find out how different swimming nude is. I'll sit there on the edge and wait for you." By the time we got to the pool the others had left. It was black as pitch and the only sounds were from the frogs in the forest pond. She slipped into the warm water, got out of her suit, and I heard it as it slapped up onto the deck. For a few minutes there was silence, and I could just barely make out her shadowy figure moving away from me. Then I couldn't see or hear her. I was beginning to worry a little when I heard a voice from the dark. "Tell me, Bonnie, what else have I missed?"

The saddest thing about inhibitions is that they are laid on innocent, healthy, *clean* material. They take root, especially if the inhibitor has value in the eyes of the material. The greater the value, the deeper the roots. Over the years these inhibitions can grow to crippling proportions and discolor all life's beautiful facets. Sometimes things get so bad that a doctor is brought in to help, usually on a one-to-one basis at exorbitant expense. The expense itself excludes most people in need. Lately, group sessions have been cropping up everywhere, and they have indeed been a godsend. In those sessions, sufferers learn that they are not alone in their problems; others have problems, and sometimes very similar problems. This at least ends their often self-imposed isolation. Occasionally, but all too seldom, these groups use the catalyst afforded by nature: the hot sun, water, soft air, the quiet night, skin exposed to the elements, which all adds up to freedom from the cares of ordinary days and from the clothing which are often indicative of the types of inhibitions being endured.

When people are ashamed of their bodies, they pull in and hold back, and neither are signs of healthy sexuality. When the muscular tension of pulling in and holding back is released, the mind seems to be released too. It happens haltingly at first and then gathers momentum. The first step is, of course, the hardest to take.

Getting back to my ten-day fitness group, I noticed that, as the days passed, bodies relaxed, rhythm improved, movement became easier, weight melted away, and people began to talk. They talked to others whom they had met only a few days before, people they really didn't know at all, if time and introductions count for anything. They talked about their most intimate secrets, about their fears and worries and the lives they lived. They shared their problems and elicited words of sympathy and encouragement from others who had had similar difficulties along the way. They relaxed and let their bodies feel the healing that nature can provide anytime she is given the chance.

By the fifth day, the sexuality of each and every one became apparent. It wasn't anything you could see with your eyes, though their sags had disappeared and they looked slimmer and stood straighter. Their muscles had relaxed and their skin was now taut. They laughed more readily and joked among themselves as many of them had not known they could. On the afternoon of the fifth day, Friday, three women who lived within driving distance asked if they might go home for the night. Now, this is a most unusual request. Women who have arranged their households so that they can be away for what might be called a vacation are rarely eager to plunge back into family responsibility. Each evening had been different, but all had been filled with good talk and lots of laughter. It should not have been easy to leave, and I wondered what lay behind the requests. When I asked the first one why she wanted to go home, she was most candid—which showed how far she had come. She said it had been ages since she had felt so warm, eager, and loving, and she wanted to go home right then and share it with her husband. I said, "Go, but be back by seven tomorrow morning." Why did I put that restriction on the trip? Because marriage is a license to make love and often what's around all the time, to take or leave alone, gets left alone. But if you have from eleven tonight until five tomorrow morning and if you find that what you have is new or renewed, you will cram a lot in, and cramming often causes heightening.

The second and third ladies were as open as the first. They were feeling something so vital and so urgent it could not be ignored. The young have it by virtue of an excess of hormones. The newly in love have it by virtue of those same triggered hormones, plus expectancy. Too often, older bodies lose it because of fatigue, hidden sickness, separation from nature, intrusion by the demanding personalities of their children. And the same deadening influences attack their mates. What these three ladies (and it turned out later, most of the others) were feeling was *desire.*

Somehow we had made an opening, and the sexuality locked inside of absolutely everyone was pouring forth. However, I was taking no chances. I called the husband of each one and told him what was coming home and to treat it with the greatest of care; it could mean a whole new way of life. Not one of them was disappointed—nor was one disappointing. Which brings me to Nell and Harry.

When I wrote that chapter about sexercise and put it in my book *How to Be Slender and Fit After Thirty,* I said many of the things I have said here. Many people bought the book for that chapter alone, and one day I got a letter from a lady who signed herself "Nell." She said she was so grateful for that chapter because it had changed her life. She had been "raised strict" and taught to think of sex as a necessary evil. Now she realized she must have missed a great deal, but worse, her beloved Harry had been cheated out of some of the best things she could have given. She had been using the sexercises for almost six months and telling herself that it was something to enjoy, right to enjoy it, and a gift to share with her love. Now she and Harry were having the time of their lives and he couldn't believe either the change in her or his great good fortune. I was delighted and wrote back what I always write when sex lives start to burn bright: "If you want children, the chances are that both your increased health, activity and desire may bring them to you. If you don't, be careful." The letter I got back was probably the most surprising of the year. She thanked me for my advice, but she didn't think she needed to worry, as she was sixty and Harry was sixty-four.

Bodies are meant to be enjoyed. Every inch of sensitive skin cries out for stimulation. Falling in love and having access to another's body brings this stimulation. It changes people's outlook on life and their feelings about everything, including themselves. When this happens, they begin to look different and you can spot a person in love quicker than you can spot a person with measles. It is also true that a body exposed to the stimulation of nature, sun, water, air, and quiet will change. If it is also given the advantage of rhythm and movement, it looks different and feels different. If you want to enhance your sexuality and release it, use what nature has to offer. You need not wait to fall in love. The love object may come to you after the fact. When you look different, feel different, and have a different outlook, you may find that the rest is easy. It won't be easy just because you are ready for it, but because that readiness can be seen by others, felt and accepted by others. Hopefully, one of them has had the same awakening.

11

How Do I Touch Thee?

While there is much to be said for eye-to-eye contact made during the first stirrings of love, and a great deal to say for the eye-to-body contact essential to encounter, touching is still the most vital means of contact we have. In our uterine beginnings we are "touched" constantly, and through touch we are made aware that we are not alone—and that it is important that we not be alone. When we are little, long before the words "I love you" have any meaning for us, those who hold us dear will say so through their fingertips and the warm palms of their hands. Their strong enfolding arms tell us that we are important to them, that we are esteemed by them, and that they love us. There isn't a word in any language that has the power of a single light touch put upon one person by another at the right time and place.

"How do I love thee? Let me count the ways . . ." could easily be translated to "How do I touch thee?" If you want to know how people feel about each other, watch them when they touch each other, whether the touch is accidental or intended. There is of course the tentative brush that *might* be accidental, except that it isn't and both parties know it. There is the firm message-giving touch of equals that accompanies spoken information and mutual admiration. You will often see the knowing, playful touch of lovers who have moments to remember and use touch that they believe to be offhand to evoke those moments. There are many ways to touch children: a pat for reassurance, a stroke for appreciation of the warmth they stir to life, the firm restraint placed on arm or shoulder when danger threatens. There is the gentle holding that goes with the greeting of old bodies who might feel pain if the embrace were vigorous.

People have a deep need to touch and to be touched, and when this need is not fulfilled their loneliness grows. Watch yourself as well as others as you move through your days. Whom do you touch and how do you touch them? Who touches you and how do they touch you? What does a firm handclasp do for your opinion of another person, and what does the limp one do? Whom do you want to touch and whom would you avoid touching if it were humanly possible? When do you feel the need to touch another? When your mood is warm and open, or when you are down?

Children (and adults) are like Yo-Yos where touch is concerned. Once children leave the maternal lap and strike out across the nursery floor, they demand the freedom to explore. However, if you watch carefully you will see that they find many reasons for coming back for a hug, a kiss, or merely a bit of grooming—all of which means being touched. Almost anything will do so long as it is warm, friendly, and personal. This may throw some light on the success of the mother who is *available* to her children during their early years. It is far from necessary or even desirable that she dance constant attendance on them every minute of the day. What they seem to need is rather some sort of home base where they can touch and be touched from time to time. This doesn't change at all when we grow up. Touching good-bye in the morning is almost never passionate (or, if so, the good-bye has to wait awhile). Touching a welcome in the evening is more reassuring than stimulating (that can wait awhile). We touch as we pass by someone we love who might be totally engrossed in a TV program. They will touch back without taking their eyes away from the screen. They don't have to; the message got through without interrupting the stimulation coming in through eyes and ears. The touch that said "I love you and I'm glad you are here at home with me tonight, I'm happy to see you enjoying yourself, you know I am near if you need me" went straight through the skin and nerves into the bio-computer. If you watch people who have been together and loved together for a long time, you will be able to see all of those messages, all given and received with no more time and effort involved than would be needed to push a button. If you watch people who have recently met and who feel something for one another, you will see that the slightest touch elicits total interest and response; everything is at attention. However, the messages are new, and while they excite, they have not formed patterns. They require thought. Watch this in yourself.

Fingertips are the most sensitive places on our bodies, and for some reason, they not only receive messages more easily than, say, the skin on our palms, they also *send* more readily and completely. Try stroking the arm of your love with your hand while you think a message and see how long it takes to get through. Then another time think the same message while stroking with your fingertips. You will be surprised. Try getting a point across to a child or an adult using words alone, and then try while resting light fingertips on the other's shoulder or arm. Long ago, I discovered that when a person in one of my classes was unable to either follow a given movement across the gym floor or stick with a rhythm, if I would take one wrist in my hand with my fingers covering the pulse, do the movement with them and *think* or *feel* it into them, it took only seconds for the most unresponsive body to follow and retain the lesson. I also learned that there were returned signals from that person which must have entered *my* bio-computer, which has been trained from infancy to react to movement, rhythm, and other people. As long as I worked with only one person and held only one wrist, we could move as one. If I tried to teach, think, and feel the movement into two people at one time via two wrists, the whole thing fell apart. I thought I was sending the same movement to both, but I had not realized that the messages coming in bespoke each individual's need and you cannot answer more than one individual's need at a time. Our wires were crossed, and the worst kind of jamming took place.

The messages sent and received between two people travel back and forth on a given wavelength, and that wavelength is peculiar to those two particular people. Touch turns the dial unerringly to the right wavelength.

If you want to reach deep into someone and speak, touch. Touch gently and easily, the way a man absent-mindedly touches the silken head of his dog. If there is anything between you, he will hear you and you will hear him.

Touch has another function besides getting the answer to "Are you for me?" or for sending messages of comfort and reassurance. Touch is a food, and without it living things wither. Life must touch life. The person who is touch-hungry is as much in need as the person who is food-hungry. Little children and young lovers put their arms around one another as they walk along. In many countries other than ours, so do adults, men with men and women with women as well as men with women. It is considered a mark of affection and healthy indeed. It says, "I like you, how nice that you are here." In America we have been at such pains to elevate sex from a healthy need to a raging want, that any signs of affection are suspect. How sad and how damaging. Not only are many people cut off from comfort and reassurance, but they are literally starved, sometimes to death.

I once knew a man who was not very young and not very attractive who went to the same bar every evening after work. He could be counted on to stand drinks all around, at least once in the hour or two he passed there. He also picked up the total tab for at least one or two people who seemed to interest him. After I had observed this off and on for several weeks, I asked him if he really liked those people who cost him most of his week's salary. "Nope, I'm just buying conversation."

Conversation-hungry, companionship-hungry, touch-hungry people have to find sustenance at any cost, and when they're touch-hungry the price can be high.

There are, of course, the professional touchers Desmond Morris talks about in his book *Intimate Behavior*: the hairdressers, manicurists, massagers, chiropractors, and many others. In too many instances these professionals are the only protection some people have against touch starvation. It is quite possible that the unseen but almost palpable drain put on male hairdressers by their yearning clients may help to account for the fact that of all professions, this one leads in heart attacks. Life needs to touch life. The fact that gardeners spend their lives doing exactly that may account at least in part for their having the fewest number of heart attacks.

Many women who have resorted to "playing the field" have very little interest in the sex act itself. What they urgently need, and are willing to pay for with their bodies if they must, is to be touched, reassured, comforted, and held. This group is not limited to singles by any means. All too many women completely surrounded by husband and family are never "touched" with warmth. Sexual intercourse does not guarantee being touched with warmth. Sometimes a neighbor lady does far more for the yearning soul by placing a comforting hand on her arm as she says she's sorry to hear that the cat got run over.

In the olden days people who were ill-suited used to stay together "for the sake of the children." They stayed together under the same roof with each other in loveless misery, and with their children, who took it all in by osmosis. In the end this fostered the loveless state on the children as well. In 1954 I read the first article I'd ever seen on *not* staying together for the sake of the children. It stated quite clearly that there were worse things than being shuttled back and forth between separated parents who were, if not deliriously happy, at least at peace. The touch coming from a person in either emotional or physical agony is like a scream for help. Children *feel* cries for help, but they rarely understand them. Disinterested adults tend to ignore such cries, and either way, little help is forthcoming. If you are in such a situation, you might try assessing your position with the full knowledge that, if you cannot touch and be touched in love and acceptance, it may be untenable. It may require an all-out effort to effect change, not just for happiness, but for your very life. Then too, if your relationships with your spouse or children seem to be lukewarm, you might want to ask yourself, "How do I touch thee?"

Each of us has a pair of hands, but most of us treat them as though they were strangers, taking them at face value and unaware of their hidden capabilities. However, biofeedback machines have revealed that man is able to transfer the heat which seems to cause splitting headaches, from his head to his finger, which doesn't suffer at all. He does it by *willing* it while monitoring his results on machines which respond to success with lights, gauges, or sounds. Each person employs different devices to effect this transfer, some sitting relaxed and thinking of nothing, others directing the heat and still others meditating on things far removed from the laboratory. Whatever means are employed, the person working to control his autonomic nervous system soon learns what it is he must do to get the desired effect. The avoidance of a debilitating headache is the reward. Those hands that are able to keep pain at bay can also be willed to transmit. Just as minds transmit rhythm and movement, hands can transmit happiness, contentment, and even healing. Healing hands seem to be attached to some of the most unlikely people, and not all of them are doctors by any means. Two of the most miraculous hands belonged to a carpenter. Such hands are usually found on people who desire to help others and who have found a way to tap their own reserves in order to send that help. Many, however, are like veins of gold hidden in the earth and unknown even to their owners. Most hands can and do transmit feelings of love without the conscious willing of these owners, but one can learn to intensify those feelings manyfold. You can too if you want to badly enough. There are no bio-feedback machines (yet) that can measure the amount of love being sent through hands, but you can check yourself from time to time. First, stop treating your hands as though they were merely tools, like a knife and fork to be used, washed, and put away until needed again. Start to watch them. The next time you are totally at peace, look at your hands. They will be still, relaxed, and quiet like your heart. If you are distressed, they will twist and clutch. If you are angry, they will close and tighten. In a way, your hands *are* you as you show yourself without intending to.

To practice sending through your hands, sit quietly and let them rest in your lap with palms up. Close your eyes and think them heavy and relaxed. You will soon be able to feel heaviness in them, and they will seem to take on a different shape and more mass, like mittens rather than separated fingers. Turn them palms down on your thighs and notice the heat coming from them, heat that you didn't feel before. Relax them even more, as though willing them to become part of your thighs. Then, without actually pressing down at all, *feel* as if your thumbs and then each individual finger were playing slow, deliberate scales on a piano keyboard. Concentrate on the tips as each receives its impulse to move, even as you send the restraining impulse. It won't be very long before you will notice tension in your shoulders; if you were actually trying to send or reinforce a message through your hands, this would interfere. Stop your scales and try to find the spot that has tightened and relax it, then begin again. It takes about ten minutes at first to achieve both total relaxation and complete concentration, but the time needed lessens with practice. After about a week of this exercise, try when you touch others to do so with just such relaxed hands and aware fingertips. Send your message either silently or aloud and see what happens. Not everyone will respond, as each has a different level of sensitivity, but some will. It is those who are listening on your wavelength who will respond, and it is those you can affect.

Touch plays a vital part in everything we do, but nothing so vital as making love. Making love is a tactile rather than a visual art, and the exquisitely sensitive fingertips not only send and receive messages, they take in information about the health and condition of the body they are touching. They report to the bio-computer on the smoothness of skin, firmness of contour, even tone of muscle. They also need press only lightly along a waistline to detect dollops of unwanted fat. They need rest for only a second on thickened, fibrositic shoulders to detect trouble. When we first started giving children the minimum muscular fitness test we could see at a glance whether they were boys or girls, tall, short, or average. Their hair and skin color were apparent, as was the state of their grooming and the care given their clothes. Training and experience taught us to interpret the way they moved, but it was by accident that we found our most reliable tool. Because we began our testing on masses of very little children, I developed the habit of holding their feet down by placing my forefinger between their ankles, my thumb and third finger on the outer sides of their feet, and the flat of my hand across their insteps. I did this so that I could control their feet better, but it was no time at all before I realized I was plugged in to something. Slide your left forefinger (if you are right-handed, otherwise reverse the procedure) over the tips of second and third fingers of your right hand. Now, with the thumb and third finger of your left hand, rub very lightly along the sides of second and third fingers of your right, only as far as the second joints. Notice the difference in sensitivity between tips and sides. Now rub the sides from the second joints right up to the slightly webbed flesh where the fingers join the hand. *There* is the most sensitive spot, and we were concentrating all our physical contact with each child onto this extremely sensitive area of ourselves. In no time at all we found we were reading through our fingers exactly the sort of *feelings* our little subjects were having. Their tensions rippled up through our hands and arms to sound very recognizable chords over the obbligato of facial expressions, movement patterns, muscle function, and occasional verbal communication. We had them pegged for minimum muscular fitness, posture and function anomalies, and emotional response, all in ninety seconds. Studies carried over months of observation by school psychologists noted the same findings.

One need not wait until a youngster starts disrupting a class to feel it coming and head it off. It is not necessary to wait until a woman escapes into a nervous breakdown before realizing that she is threatened. Long before a person's total organization falls into either temporary or permanent confusion and despair, the body sends out thousands of signals calling for help. We may not have the trained ears that hear or eyes that see with knowledge, but everyone has hands that can feel longing, anger, and anxiety just as readily as they can feel love. But you don't feel anything at all unless you are willing to touch as a kind of question and touch again as the answer requires—with gentleness, caring, and love.

12

You Are What You Eat . . . Even in Bed

There is a not-so-funny joke around. It is said that one-half of America goes to bed hungry; they are all on diets. This is a pretty sad joke in today's world of shortages, energy crises, and worldwide starvation. It wouldn't sound funny to the man in Calcutta whose children go to bed hungry because there's nothing to eat. We might be a little less smug if we really understood that a goodly number of our people who are not on diets and who don't feel hungry are living with severe deficiencies that affect their bodies, brains, sex lives, emotional stability, and happiness. In India there just isn't enough to go around. In America, land of plenty, what's going around isn't enough, but the lack isn't in quantity, it is in quality and substance.

When you were in school, there was probably a class in sex education. None of the kids learned anything they didn't know already, but the teacher often did. The book was clear and concise. It dealt with SEX in capital letters, and you may have wondered how it was possible to make such an interesting subject so boring. Over the years, you have probably come to realize that it seems to be one of the functions of school to make vital, exciting, valuable material as dull, uninteresting and devoid of any connection with the students as possible. It was usually the same way in classes dealing with nutrition.

During those sleepy afternoons when you studied about "nutrition" (two credits or you wouldn't have been there in the first place), you wrote notes to your neighbor, dreamed about the malted you'd have with your special friend after school, and you drew pictures of the vegetables they were discussing, with faces, arms, and legs. You "learned" that milk made teeth and bones. So what! You already had teeth and bones. Vegetables had different colors. Big deal! You knew that in first grade. You heard lectures on minerals, vitamins, carbohydrates, fats, and proteins—ho-hum. All those things had *something* to do with the alimentary canal, blood, tissues, glands and stuff, but they had nothing to do with you. You memorized the names the same way you did Tiberius, Caligula, Claudius, and Nero, and right after the quiz you promptly forgot them, though you did remember that butter was a fat, steak a protein, a potato was a carbohydrate, and salad was roughage with vitamins. You were even served some information about the effects of alcohol on the human body, and drug addiction was decried as destructive. However, nobody mentioned sugar addiction or pointed out that you were already, like most Americans, well hooked. How come? Here's how come.

Well before you got teeth, you were served sugar in your cereal if not in your formula. It was added to your applesauce and pureed apricots. Why? Because your mother would not have bought the brand that tasted a little sour; she tasted all your food first and she liked sugar in food. Then, your rewards for good behavior, as well as the stoppers for your screaming mouth, were cookies, candies, and pretty soon, gum. Sugar was added to your orange juice, and soon you preferred chocolate milk to the white kind.

A check with most school kids' breakfasts would yield up bushels of sugar-crusted flakes, mountains of sweet rolls, rivers of cocoa, chocolate milk, and sweet fruit drinks. A similar watch put on their lunches is no more encouraging as they swap brownies, cake slices, cookies, and candy bars. When they go home, you can be certain that their first move after turning on the TV (if it isn't on already) will be to the freezer for an ice-cream stick. They'll skip the beans, carrots, or turnips at supper, but have a second piece of pie. While they are doing their homework they will go through at least two Cokes (which may be why they are still awake at eleven) a box of Mallowmars and four Lorna Doones.

Quite possibly you may have heard that sugar wasn't good for you—"Never give the dog candy, dear, it's very bad for dogs"—and maybe your mother was the kind who kept repeating, like a TV commercial, "Brush after meals . . . brush after meals." Again, so what! For again it had nothing to do with you. Occasionally it would be called to your attention that the intelligence levels of children being raised under conditions of semistarvation were low. But again, so what! That didn't mean anything to you either. You lived in America, the richest country in the world, where there was plenty of food. The starving kids of Africa and India were just pictures in the *National Geographic.* How strange that no one ever told you that one of the reasons you sometimes had trouble taking in and retaining information might have been due to the fact that kids right here in America have starved brains and that, yes, you were one of them. At no time were you ever given any vital, exciting, *disturbing* information that made you want to look into the food on *your* table. Well, here is some vital, exciting, and disturbing information that may jolt you into just that. It may change your entire life.

If you are a woman in love, you should know that you can keep your man alive or kill him off in short order by what you put in front of him at mealtimes and by the amount of information you can get into his head that will affect his luncheon habits. Statistics say that even if you and your husband are the same age, you will be a widow for eight years. It would certainly be worth the effort to cut that figure down. Widowhood isn't "merry" at all.

If you are a man in love, your ability to make love

long and well will depend in large part on the health of your body and mind, and that depends in large part on what you eat, as does the length of your life itself. Whichever sex you are, your level of sexuality also depends on your health, which depends on what does or does not go into your mouth. Why do you suppose athletes sit at training tables, dancers haunt health-food stores, and that actresses, models, and other assorted beauties who live or die (professionally speaking) by their appearance are so careful about their food? It's because they know full well what your teacher failed to teach you, that both looks and physical performance (any kind) depend on nutrition. To be any good at selecting food that is nutritious in America, the land where the picture on the box has more value than the contents, you need to be a very well-informed and very suspicious person.

Let's start with bread, because it is by a change in the processing of flour for bread that we can locate the sudden rise in heart attacks. That fatally silent and all too often killing disease was virtually unknown before the early 1900's. Then a new milling process for grains became popular. This process removed all the most valuable parts of those grains (animals now get them in their foods) and left devitalized white flour behind for people—*you.* The white flour was then bleached by gas to make it whiter and presumably "richer," softer, and therefore supposedly "tastier." If you have ever tasted bread baked from freshly stone-ground flour, you know that the insipid, formless, spongy breads so highly advertised (and it's the advertising you pay for) for their "enrichment" and "body-building" properties have only one adjective in their advertisements which really applies—"softer." And softer is a bad word. American "store-bought" bread is not what the poet had in mind when he spoke of "A loaf of bread, a jug of wine, and thou." It doesn't deserve the name and is palatable only under a spread. Fifty years later, at just about the time we began to realize how life-preserving those lost nutrients were, the true nature of our danger surfaced in the form of thousands upon thousands of heart attacks. In order to quiet warning voices, the manufacturers put back token amounts of those nutrients. A word picture for their action is this: you go out to the bus stop and are mugged. Your wallet, watch, and gold chain are stolen. As the thief disappears down a dark alley, he turns and throws fifty cents at your feet, whispering, "Don't go away mad."

Now, let's take sugar, since it too plays an ominous role and you probably ingest a great deal of it whether you know it or not. The source of sugar is cane, and there's nothing wrong with it until it is processed, at which time *all* nutrients are destroyed. This guarantees the product almost limitless shelf life, which, while helpful to the supermarket owner, is not so good for you. That sugar isn't merely worthless, it's downright dangerous.

When you were in school, you were sure (you may still be) that sugar provided "quick energy." That's nonsense. Sugar requires a greater percentage of the body's energy to utilize it than the energy it provides, thereby causing *energy debt*. It also interferes with your vitamin balance. If your regular diet provided all the B vitamins necessary for health and everything was perking right along, the addition of a very small amount of sugar could cause a vitamin deficiency. If you are a sugar addict (Cokes, cake, candy, ice cream, soda pop, pies, sweet rolls, doughnuts, tarts), you do that sort of thing to yourself all the time. Vitamin-B deficiencies are quite common in opulent America.

You probably did learn in school that if you ate a lot of candy you got cavities, but nobody ever told you that the trouble caused by the sugar in your mouth was the least of it. The sugar in your body is also destructive. It slows down the movement of the fluids *within* the teeth. This weakens them, laying them open to decay.

Perhaps at this moment you are feeling quite smug; you don't even like all those sugary things, you are the exception and are consequently perfectly safe. Guess again.

Sugar has been added to just about everything on your supermarket shelves. There is as much as two tablespoons in a *small* glass of fruit-ade, gingerale, colas, cider, gelatin dessert, ice cream, puddings, canned fruit, or one single cookie (there's no such thing as one single cookie). Not for kicks but for the sake of your sex life, take a magnifying glass with you to the supermarket. Go right down any aisle between cans, jars, bottles, and boxes and check the ingredients listed for sugar (dextrose, maltose, or sucrose). Unless you are over in the Lestoil section, you'll find almost nothing free of sugar, including tomatoes and soups. If you have a garden and grow your own tomatoes, you know very well that they don't require sugar, nor does soup.

Oh, well, what's a little sugar, a little tooth decay, and a little vitamin deficiency, you may ask. Not much if you don't mind a little atherosclerosis thrown in. Excess sugar consumption is statistically associated with atherosclerosis and heart attacks. Autopsies performed on twenty-one-year-old boys who died in front-line action in Korea revealed that 77 percent of them already had gross evidence of the disease. A similar study done in Vietnam points up, as do our muscle tests, that things haven't improved over the years. All the front-line casualties examined suffered in varying degrees from the disease. How old are *you*?

Next time you go shopping, look into the baskets of old people with the understanding that the digestion of elders is not as good as it once was and therefore they need *more* nutritious food than they used to. Because of the sharp reduction in income accompanying retirement for most people, those baskets represent tragedies on wheels. They have had to forgo steaks, roasts, eggs, and other nutritious foods and replace them with carbohydrates, which are filling but of questionable value in America. In other lands where our milling process is not used, tortillas, spaghetti, cereals, bread, and similar products still retain life-giving properties. Now, think in terms of the diet *forced* on old people, then of their forgetfulness, their occasional crankiness, irritability, lack of spring and balance, their fatigue and their aches and pains. Did you know that every one of those problems also goes with poor nutrition?

Next, what do you know about vitamins other than that some doctors say they are important while still others claim that if you have a balanced diet you don't need them? The first thing to know about them is that they can't be used *instead of food.* All too many people go on crash diets feeling perfectly safe and well-nourished because they take one of those magical all-in-one-once-a-day vitamin pills. Their maintenance, growth, and repair are as fully covered as their bodies would be if they went streaking across Madison Square Garden. This is what you need to know about vitamins: when they are present in your cells they bring about certain helpful processes, one of which is to assist in the digestion and utilization of nourishing foods. In other words, vitamins are like factory workers; they can put the car together, but first they need the right materials.

There are two kinds of vitamins: water-soluble and fat-soluble. Good sources of fat-soluble vitamins are liver and eggs. Incidentally, all that flap about eggs raising your cholesterol level has just about evaporated, and you will see why a little further on. Good sources of water-soluble vitamins are fruits and vegetables. However, you already knew that. What you may not have known is that water-soluble vitamins will leach right out of the vegetables and salads when left to soak in water. Most of the good in frozen vegetables will be lost to you if you permit them to thaw before cooking, and therein lies one of the sad things about supermarkets. You pay top dollar for frozen vegetables, and quite often they have been allowed to thaw and then been refrozen. One thing more. Cook in very little water or steam your vegetables. In both cases, don't overcook, and be sure to keep the lid on tight to prevent oxidation. *Don't throw out the water left from cooking;* valuable minerals will be lost. Put it in the refrigerator, and when you want a cup of broth, use your vegetable water to add to the broth square or package.

If you take your vitamins in tablet or capsule form and then wash them down with a glass of water, only the water-soluble vitamins will dissolve. If there was no fat in your stomach (your egg, bacon, butter, cheese, or fish), the fat-soluble vitamins like E will waltz right on by, not only wasting your money, but giving you a false sense of security.

When tempted to rely on a single vitamin, let's say Vitamin C, please understand that vitamins are not soloists. They work together in teams, and they also work with minerals. Taking one while omitting all the others is like trying to fight a battle with plenty of tanks but no gasoline, or with a sufficiency of guns but no ammunition.

If you want good information on vitamins, ask a doctor, but choose your doctor with great care. Years ago when I started exercise classes, most people were as ignorant about exercises and their own bodies as they are today about vitamins and their own bodies. Many asked me if they should consult a doctor before signing up. I always said by all means they should if they felt the need, but to select a doctor with square shoulders, a flat abdomen, and a tight seat. That would mean he knew something about exercise and would probably be in favor of it. If they went to a man who looked like a tired pear, he probably would not. So before you make your appointment with the doctor, find out if he approves of vitamins. If he does, go ahead. Here is what a few doctors think.

Dr. Granville F. Knight, M.D., FACA, in Santa Monica, California, says, "Food processing and preparation result in the loss of large amounts of important vitamins and minerals. Selection of a good diet, including the avoidance of empty-calorie foods such as sugar, white flour, and polished rice, is important, but it is not enough.

Supplements of vitamins A, C, B-complex, D, and E with emphasis on desiccated liver and powdered yeast are essential for good health."

Fine, you may say, but how much? On many of today's food packages, most notably cereals, you will find an announcement to the effect that the contents provide all the minimum daily requirements recommended by the FDA (federal Food and Drug Administration). If that requirement was really enough, as the wording implies, you wouldn't have a worry in the world after eating your bowl of All, Whiskers, or Catch-22, but is it enough?

George Prastka, M.D., Costa Mesa, California, says, "Shambles have been made out of the FDA's *Minimum Daily Requirements and Recommended Daily Allowances* of various vitamins and minerals by countless scientific studies. This is because there is a tremendous variation in the range of the requirements of so-called normal persons. Indeed, we have yet to discover the optimum amounts of these substances for the human body. This is even more true of the individual. One person may require perhaps one thousand times more of a given nutrient than another, *due in many cases to the problem he may have in assimilating it.*" (Italics mine.)

O.K., you say, but how much is enough? H. L. Newbold, M.D., of New York, says, "No one knows what are your requirements for optimal health. My best advice is to take very large amounts of all the water-soluble vitamins plus brewer's yeast."

Fine, you say, but how much is too much? A. Hoffer, M.D., Ph.D., of Saskatchewan, says, "The body can deal with an excess of vitamins and minerals much more effectively than it can deal with a deficiency. In other words, more than is required does much less harm than too little, as the body handles an excess by simply getting rid of it. The water-soluble vitamins are not harmful in quantities far above the minimum daily requirements of the FDA, as they are easily thrown off by the body if they are not needed."

Vitamin A and Sexuality

Vitamin-A deficiency is borderline in America, but it is quite possible for one of you to be on the wrong side of the border. Vitamin A protects the "specialized epithelial surfaces"—that would be the tissues in your mouth, lungs, glands, your digestive tract, and in fact all the protective covering of your skin. In those few words you can see that if you were deficient in vitamin A, your sexuality level would be lowered severely. The genitals are also "specialized epithelial surfaces."

Here are some sources of vitamin A, starting with the item contributing most per serving. Fresh calf's liver. Sautéed and served with crisp bacon, it is delicious. Overcook and it turns to gray leather. Either way, a serving of liver gives you about 20,000 I.U.'s (International Units).

If you prefer vegetables because you can't stand liver, spinach comes in at 14,000 I.U.'s, dandelion greens at 12,500, and chard or beet tops at 12,000 per serving. Escarole, kale, sweet potatoes, and tomato puree provide 10,000 each. Between 5,000 and 7,000 units are found in onions, turnips, turnip greens, tomatoes and tomato juice. But possibly the best sources of all are halibut and cod-liver oil. (You can get cod-liver oil in health-food stores in perle form—pearl-shaped capsules.)

Vitamin E and Sexuality

E is just about the most controversial of all the vitamins. It is certainly the most maligned and least understood. It does have the advantage of being known as the sex vitamin because it has a beneficial effect on the hormones necessary for reproduction. But it does even more. It is a prime antioxidant, and if you love hamburgers, french fries, hot dogs, and potato chips, you'd better know what an antioxidant is. E inhibits reactions caused by oxygen in the blood. Oxygen turns fat rancid, and rancid fats damage the red-cell membranes.

If you are deficient in vitamin E, you are far more susceptible to stress—any kind of stress, from real sorrow to a nervous interview. If you are taking medication containing iron (and there are several on TV which you are urged to take daily, whether you need them or not), you should be aware that ferric chloride destroys E, and you will need to replenish your natural supply as well as supplement it.

The new milling process destroyed the nutrients in flour by removing the hull of the wheat and discarding it. The hull is particularly rich in Vitamin E, and there went a marvelous source of it! E should be considered when you think about heart-attack prevention.

E helps prevent blood from clotting abnormally. It also strengthens the small blood vessels, which in turn improves circulation.

Vitamin E is necessary for good muscle tone, as athletes have known for years. Your athletic feats do not necessarily take place on the court or course, of course. A deficiency can cause muscle cramps, especially at night . . . and where would *that* leave you?

E is a marvelous skin conditioner. If you want yours to look its best, don't waste money on the highly advertised Magical Nostrums. They merely keep the skin from *losing* moisture, while E replaces it. It helps in healing and prevents scarring, which should be important to anyone suffering from acne, facial injury, or burns. Ever since hearing from Nell and Harry, I have remembered that years have very little to do with limiting sex, and so I am sure that some of you will need this information about vitamin E. Many recent studies point to the destruction of fat by oxidation as a prime cause of cell deterioration, the same sort of cell deterioration that causes aging. E should certainly be on the shopping list of anyone over forty. Age is one thing, aging quite another.

Processing and heat both destroy vitamin E in foods, so you will have to make sure that you are getting a sufficient amount. The best natural sources are wheat-germ oil, mackerel, soya oil, and refined corn oil. It is reported that E, like C, is harmless even when taken in large amounts, but people with high blood pressure should consult their doctors before embarking on a program of vitamin supplementation. For that matter, people with high blood pressure should consult their doctors before embarking on most new things.

Vitamin B-Complex and Sexuality

Without the B-complex vitamins your body can't do anything at all with the food you eat, no matter how carefully you select it or how much you pay for it. These vitamins play a key role in converting all the fats, proteins, and carbohydrates to your use and they are very clannish. Not only do they work together in your behalf, but they can't do a proper job unless they are *all* there. Leave one out and the others falter. Then you are not only poorly provided for, but susceptible to disease. And I'll bet no teacher of nutrition ever told you that adding junk food to your diet subtracts from the ability of the B-complex vitamins to process valuable nutrients, for the vitamins must divide their talents between processing food with value and food with none—and that's a waste of talent. You see, food with value *brings* nutrients to the party. Junk food doesn't come with a single house gift, but is every bit as avid at the banquet table. The B that *should* go to work for you is sidetracked into taking care of the kind of house guests you'd never invite twice if you understood what they were doing. Cap that thought with the fact that one-half the national diet is made up of junk food. Just how "national" are you?

The B vitamins are the ones you can cook to death over a slow fire. Don't expect any to survive in the stew; you'll have to have a salad to go with it. You can throw them out with the vegetable water you very carefully kept to a minimum and you can poison them with baking soda, which your grandmother used to keep the peas bright green. Since they do their best work when in each other's company, you can be sure of their cooperation by taking three tablespoons of yeast every day—you'll get used to it. If you take it in orange juice at breakfast or with milk midmorning or midafternoon, it doesn't taste half bad. Yeast is a lot like the pill; once it's down, you don't have to worry about something else cropping up.

It might be a good thing to know a little about each of the B vitamins because it is with those vitamins that the food processors try to lull you into thinking their products have value. It is their names you will see listed on the so-called "enriched" foods. However, the processors will not be able to con you if you bear in mind that the B vitamins must interact; a product that claims to provide you with an extra boost of vitamin B_2 isn't going to boost anything unless all the other B vitamins are also in the food, ready to trigger each other off.

Thiamine (B_1)

Without thiamine you could contract beriberi, which causes stiff ankles, leg pains, numbness, and tingling in the toes. Paralysis can set in and your heart will act up. If you had a mild thiamine deficiency, you could then develop a mild case of beriberi with milder symptoms, but still the same symptoms. You can also feel terribly depressed, irritable, and tired. It also affects learning, should you still be a student. When you are pregnant, thiamine helps with morning sickness, as does a diet high in protein. If you hate the dentist because your pain threshold is low, take thiamine. It also speeds healing and lessens the chatter after the Novocain wears off. If your work is physical, take thiamine. If you smoke or take a few drinks at the end of the day, thiamine.

Thiamine is in almonds, asparagus, bacon, barley, beef heart, brewer's yeast, calf's liver, cashews, cornmeal, ham, lentils, limas, pecans, lean pork, rye flour, soybeans, soy flour, spareribs, wheat bran, and wheat germ.

Riboflavin (B_2)

This may be our greatest vitamin deficiency, which is too bad, since it is essential for the normal functioning of the gastrointestinal tract. Cooking is not its enemy, but alcohol, baking soda, and daylight are. The first signs of riboflavin deficiency are cracked lips (mothers take note), purple tongue (older people take note), burning and dryness of the eyes, and sensitivity to light (all you wearers of dark glasses take note). Alcoholics often show marked signs of riboflavin deficiency, but so do social drinkers. Where can you find your protection?

Brewer's yeast, cheese, eggs, hickory nuts, kidneys, limas, liver, dried milk, peanut butter (get it in a health-food store—no additives), soybeans, soy flour, wheat, wheat bran, wheat germ, wheat hearts, and whey—which is especially good (health-food store).

Pyridoxine (B_6)

Pyridoxine is an antihistamine which works against the toxic substance histamine—and what's that? People have been taking antihistamines for years to combat allergies but they rarely know what histamine they are anti. It is putrefied amino acids, and if there isn't a clean-up department to protect you against the accumulation of such putrefaction, allergies take over. That should be of interest to those of you who *think* you have a "sinus drip" or *know* you are allergic to cats.

One doesn't often think of vitamins in connection with starting babies, but a lack of this one can result in a lack of start. Other unpleasantness related to a lack of sufficient pyridoxine are diarrhea, hemorrhoids, eczema, ulcers, nausea, and nervous disorders. Good sources are brewer's yeast (again), cabbage, limas, liver, peanuts, peas, molasses, and sweet potatoes.

Cobalamin (B_{12})

This particular vitamin combats anemia, neuritis, diabetes, and even some forms of psychoses. And where lies your protection? Fish, kidneys, liver (again), meat, and milk.

Niacin

A lack of niacin can make life absolutely intolerable for a human being, his family, and his co-workers. It can be what causes people to say "What's eating *him*?" or "Who does he think *he* is?" or even "Who needs *her*?" It can result in a complete personality change. The least unpleasant symptom is inflammation of the mouth. Others are digestive disorders, diarrhea, abdominal pain, and of course, depression.

Sources are the same as for thiamine. You can find additional help in beef heart, brewer's yeast, chicken, desiccated liver (sounds awful but comes in nearly tasteless tablets at the health-food store), mackerel, mushrooms, peanut butter, pork, salmon, swordfish, turkey, veal, wheat bran, and whole-wheat flour. When you think in terms of whole wheat, don't include commercially baked whole-wheat bread. For the most part there is no more *whole* wheat in that type than in any other.

Pantothenic Acid

Pantothenic acid relieves peripheral neuritis, and a deficiency often causes fatigue, fainting, and a disturbed pulse rate. There are three symptoms your school nurse saw in abundance: cracked nails (which is one reason for biting them), depression (often called a mood), and susceptibility to infection. Do you have a lot of colds?

Protection lies with the now familiar eggs, liver, peanuts, peas, wheat germ, and yeast.

Biotin

This particular vitamin is needed in order to produce fat and to combat skin rashes and eczema. Help is to be found in beef liver, cauliflower, cow peas, lamb liver, sardines, soybeans, soy flour, yeast, and rice, unpolished, which means you can't cook it in five minutes but must buy it at a health-food store and cook it properly for least twenty minutes.

Inositol

Inositol is responsible for the production of lecithin, a *food* that is partially responsible for the burning of cholesterol. It helps keep the arteries clear. A deficiency can lead to high levels of cholesterol and blood sugar and to coronary disease. Suggested sources are beef brains and hearts, cabbage, dried limas, soybeans, wheat germ and yeast. Lecithin comes in granules, perls, or capsules at health-food stores.

Many people throw up their hands at the mention of such things as beef hearts, kidneys, or brains. Don't. Get Adelle Davis' book *Let's Cook It Right* and discover what a little imagination can do with unfamiliar things. Beef-heart stew is excellent, and brains in bacon rings are a gourmet specialty.

Folic Acid (Pteroyglutamic Acid)

This one has a tremendous responsibility, as it aids in the reproduction of red blood cells. It too prevents inflammation of the mouth. Dentists are often the first to know when you suffer from a vitamin deficiency or stress. If anyone you know is nursing a baby or plans to, folic acid is a must.

All dark green vegetables are high in folic acid, but don't overcook them. Other sources are asparagus, beef, broccoli, cantaloupe, chicken, lettuce, limas, liver, oysters, salmon, watermelon, wheat germ, and yeast.

PABA (Para-Aminobenzoic Acid)

One of the reasons you feel so awful when you take antibiotics, which often make you feel you would prefer the disease to the cure, is that antibiotics have the ability to move into your body-house and kick the legitimate tenant PABA right out the door. Your PABA may have been in fine supply before you were given the antibiotics, but once the two begin to vie for *lebensraum,* PABA loses and you have a deficiency. Result: digestive disorders and nervousness—and give that last one four stars. PABA is an excellent skin ointment; it prevents aging skin and wrinkles and is essential for healthy shining hair. When you see dry, lifeless hair, particularly on the aged and on teenage boys, wonder about their diets. Do they contain bran, eggs, milk, molasses, rice, wheat germ, whole wheat, and yeast?

Choline

Choline is needed in the manufacture of the amino acid tyrosine, and tyrosine is essential to thyroid hormones, which are necessary to weight control. Perhaps you are beginning to see that your body is something like the little old lady in the nursery rhyme, the one who wanted to get home before dark. She hit the dog, the dog bit the cat, and the cat scratched the rat, and so on until everybody got going in the right direction. Your body is made up of teams within teams. Let a couple of players call in sick or simply stay away, and you are in trouble.

Choline deficiency can lead to a weight problem, muscle weakness, and muscle scarring. It too is effective in lowering blood cholesterol levels. If you plan to nurse a baby, choline is a must. You will find it in calf's liver, eggs, kidneys, peas, pork, snap beans, soybeans, wheat germ, and yeast.

B_{15} (Pangamic Acid)

This is a very important vitamin if you live or work in the city. It protects against carbon-monoxide poisoning. It also aids in the metabolism of fat and the assimilation of oxygen and it stimulates both the glandular and nervous systems. Found in all the foods that are sources for B vitamins.

With your perhaps newly acquired knowledge about the sources of the vital B vitamins, you should view with some alarm the diets of teenagers who go to school without breakfast, have a quick hamburger with Coke and fries for lunch, a couple of candy bars and another Coke at about four, a pickup supper between basketball practice and homework—and a final insult, a frozen pizza and one more Coke before bed. Those kids feel awful. They think awful is normal, and therefore anything must be better than "normal." Different from "normal" is "high." We keep looking for complicated reasons for drug addiction. Perhaps we should look in the kitchen.

Vitamin C and Sexuality

Vitamin C is the busiest, most talented jack-of-all-trades in the whole vitamin family. While most animals can manufacture their own supply within their own bodies, man cannot, and it is all too often in short supply. Irwin Stone, a biochemist in San Jose, California, says, "Lack of vitamin C has contributed to more deaths, sickness, and misery than any other factor in man's long history. Modern evidence indicates that optimal needs for full health are closer to five thousand milligrams than sixty milligrams." (*National Health Federation Bulletin*, July–August 1973.)

Those most likely to suffer from C deficiency are children, dieters, alcoholics, heavy smokers, old folks, teenagers, and those who eat on the run. Dr. R. Klenner of Riedsville, North Carolina, says, "I recommend one thousand milligrams of vitamin C for all my patients for each year of age until they are ten years old and then taking ten thousand milligrams a day. I advise them to maintain that level as they grow older and to increase if necessary. My personal intake is eighteen thousand milligrams a day." (*National Health Federation. Bulletin*, July–August 1973.)

Vitamin C cannot be stored and must be replaced constantly *all day long*. It is our major fighter against infection, but no one can predict when exposure to infection will take place. If you are counting on your morning orange juice to do your fighting for you, it may fall short by four in the afternoon when the man next to you coughs in your face. If you had one cigarette after drinking that orange juice, forget it; you wiped out your protection right then.

The person going into a hospital for an operation usually checks his health insurance very carefully, cleans up his desk, and packs what the hospital won't provide, his toothbrush. The hospital rarely provides vitamin C either, yet it is known as an incomparable aid in recovery. E. Cheraskin, M.D. at the University of Alabama, says, "Clinical tests clearly show that the ingestion of vitamin C in amounts greater than generally recommended significantly speeds wound healing."* Harold Stone, DDS, La Habra, California, says, "One gram of vitamin C per hour (for approximately eight hours) prevents mouth infections following extractions and also increases the integrity of the tissues involved. In using vitamin C for the last thirty-five years we have not had to use antibiotics, which are harmful to the bacterial flora of the intestinal tract."*

C is located in the white blood cells, which not only

* *National Health Federation Bulletin*, July–August 1973.

fight infection in general but viruses in particular. It should be considered (although no one has mentioned it very loudly) that since some cancers are caused by viruses and vitamin C is the sworn enemy of viruses, we might have a champion we are overlooking.

C prevents the breakage of the small capillary cells which can cause hemorrhages under the skin. It prevents the formation of kidney stones by neutralizing the alkaline solution required for their formation. It also carries hydrogen into the body, aids in burning food, healing wounds, fighting germs, and in the assimilation of iron. Why take an iron tonic and forget its assimilator?

Linus Pauling, the Nobel prizewinner at Stanford University in Palo Alto, California, says in his book *The Common Cold* that taking up to ten thousand milligrams of C a day will prevent and cure the common cold. He has also said that a tenfold increase in the daily intake can lead to a higher level of intelligence. (Did you ever wonder how much vitamin C the children in the Head Start Centers get?) That tenfold increase will also lead to a feeling of well-being, physically and mentally.

Every form of stress, from hard physical work, consumption of additives in food, air pollution, heat, cold, noise, mental or emotional tension, smoking, the ingestion of alcohol or drugs (even the prescribed kind), calls for a goodly supply of vitamin C.

Sources of vitamin C are alfalfa meal, almonds, apple juice, asparagus, bananas, blueberries, cabbage, cantaloupe, carrots, celery, chard, chicken livers, collards, cranberries, currants, and citrus fruits. The peels from those fruits have twice as much C as the fruits themselves, but you have to reckon with the fact that the fruits are often dyed for eye appeal and the danger from the chemical dyes outweighs the advantages. Endive, grapes, milk, parsley, peas, peppers, radishes, spinach, sprouts, strawberries, tangerines, tomatoes, turnip greens, watercress, and watermelon also supply vitamin C.

Vitamin P (Bioflavonoids)

To get the most from your oranges and grapefuit, don't squeeze the juice or segment them. Peel them and eat the whole thing. That white inner lining and the pulp contain the bioflavonoids, or vitamin P. This vitamin helps prevent the passage of serum protein through the capillary walls and thus prevents edema.

Vitamin F (known as essential fatty acids)

Vitamin F helps maintain the lubrication and resilience of the cells. It is necessary for normal glandular activity, particularly that of the adrenals, which play such an important part in your sex life. F protects against X-rays and it is questionable whether people forced by disease to undergo a course in X-ray therapy are ever even told about the effects of this vitamin. It assists with the assimilation of calcium, helps keep the skin healthy, and prevents allergies and sinus infections.

Sources are cold-pressed unrefined vegetable oils, linseed oil, safflower oil, soybean oil, and sunflower oil.

Vitamin D and Sexuality

This is the vitamin your teachers told you was for bones and teeth, which was all right with you. You drank milk, and milk was a source of D. As far as you were concerned, it was those milkless kids in India who got rickets, which was what you got if you didn't drink milk. But let's look at sexuality. If your supply of D is low, you will suffer from muscle weakness, low stamina, instability in your nervous system, muscle twitches, and cramps. Prevention of such misery is to be found in eggs, fish, fish liver, oils, and meat. Don't forget your sunbaths with oil on your skin, and don't wash it off for four hours. That's how long absorption takes.

Minerals and Sexuality

There is a wide variety of minerals, and you know what they say about variety being the spice of life. Consider that and then consider what minerals do for you and for your sexuality. They contribute to the body's energy supply and use, proper functioning of the body's organs, and the health of the bones, teeth, hair and complexion—all important contributions to one's overall health and appearance and, therefore, to one's sexuality.

Back in your nutrition class, minerals boiled down to one—iron. That would be like saying to a man from Mars, "The human body is comprised of a leg." Without minerals, the vitamins couldn't do their jobs and, as with the B vitamins, you need some of every one of them.

Calcium and Sexuality

Calcium cannot function without the presence of vitamins A, C, and D. If you knew anything about it in school, it was that it went into teeth and bones. Fine as far as it goes, but as you have said before, you already *have* teeth and bones, and what else is new? Probably the most important thing you need to know in this age of stress, crisis, and trouble is that calcium helps you combat stress and, in combination with magnesium (health-food store), it can act as a very efficient tranquilizer.

If your level of calcium drops, you become tired, which may again explain the need some people feel for the "lift" that goes with a "Benny" (Benzedrine pill). The difference between popping a "Benny" and drinking a glass of milk is the way you feel four hours later when the pill has worn itself (and you) out.

Without sufficient calcium, nerve impulses cannot be transported from one part of the body to the other. Try to keep remembering that although sex may begin in your head, it goes other places too—compliments of the nervous system! Souces are easy to find, even in our nonfood food stores, and include just about anything in the dairy department. Incidentally, a yogurt is much better than an Eskimo Pie. Calcium is also to be found in green vegetables, and the best source is bone meal (health-food store).

Phosphorus and Sexuality

Phosphorus is present in every cell. It converts oxidative energy to cell work and influences the synthesis of proteins, fats, and carbohydrates. The solid part of your brain is made up of phosphorized fats, which gradually increase as your nervous system matures. Good sources are veal bone meal and chalaza (health-food store).

Iron and Sexuality

You are asked by Madison Avenue to believe that iron is necessary if women wish to look young (and do good housework)! Actually it is found in the cells of *both* men and women and is necessary for the red-colored substance called hemoglobin. Since it carries oxygen to the brain as well as everywhere else, a lack of it may interfere with memory, learning, efficiency on the job, advancement, and self-image. Good sources are desiccated liver (remember, tablets), eggs, leafy vegetables, molasses (instead of sugar), and sun-dried raisins.

Iodine and Sexuality

Most of the iodine in your system is to be found in your thyroid gland. It stimulates and regulates both metabolism and energy. A deficiency can easily cause a weight problem and sluggishness, and neither problem is helpful to your self-image. Sources are dulse and kelp (health-food store), and onions and vegetables grown in iron-rich soil.

Sodium and Sexuality

Sodium is almost as busy as vitamin C. It helps maintain the normal water balance between the cells and fluids. It provides your muscles with the strength to contract to nerve stimulation, which it also influences. Without it the pelvic tilt couldn't happen. Sodium is a great team member that works with potassium to maintain the favorable acid-base factor. It teams with chlorine to improve the condition of both blood and lymph. It helps change carbohydrates into fat, processes amino acids, and guards against heat stroke and muscle cramps in hot environments. Sources are beets, carrots, chard, dandelion greens, poultry, and seafood.

Potassium and Sexuality

It works with phosphate to send oxygen to the brain, and with sodium to regulate your heartbeat. It stimulates the kidneys and feeds muscles. Sources are blackstrap molasses, chicory, citrus fruits, figs, mint, green peppers, and watercress.

Magnesium and Sexuality

Magnesium has functions similar to those of calcium. Dr. Michael Walczak says, "Magnesium activates more enzymes in the body than any other mineral. Among other things, it is also intimately involved in the storage of sugar as glycogen in the liver, and in its release into the blood for energy. Yet the so-called "balanced diet" provides only about 25 percent of the amount required for good health. (*National Health Federation Bulletin*, July–August 1973.) Magnesium and calcium in combination are found in dolomite tablets, which have a remarkably calming effect. Many athletes use them before stressful tournaments, and ordinary cowards are eased through a dentist's appointment with a few dolomite tablets. Other sources of magnesium are almonds, apples, celery, figs, grapefruit, lemons, nuts, seeds, wild rice, and yellow corn.

Copper and Sexuality

It is absolutely essential that copper be present in the body if iron is to be converted into hemoglobin. Sources are almonds, dried beans, beef and calf's liver, eggs, dried peas, shrimp, and whole wheat.

Sulfur and Sexuality

Sulfur is a part of the amino acids that builds tissues and cells and works with vitamins. It causes the liver to secrete bile and is important for a good complexion and healthy hair. Sources are dried beans, lean beef, cabbage, fish, eggs, and sprouts.

Silicon and Sexuality

Silicon joins other minerals to build bones, and it forms tooth enamel. Sources are buckwheat products, carrots, liver, mushrooms, and tomatoes.

Zinc and Sexuality

Combined with phosphorus, zinc aids in respiration, helping the tissues to take in oxygen and expel carbon dioxide. The insulin in your body cannot function without the presence of zinc, nor will the storage of glycogen be efficiently carried out. It is a constituent of the male reproductive fluid and aids in the manufacture of male hormones—*those hormones that are responsible for erotic excitation in both males and females.* Major source, liver.

Manganese and Sexuality

Manganese combines with phosphorus to build strong bones. It is needed for good digestion, healthy nerves, and the formation of milk in nursing mothers.

Sources are beets, eggs, *unmilled* grains, green leaves, and peas.

Chlorine and Sexuality

Chlorine stimulates the liver as a waste filter, cleans out toxic substances, helps in the production of hydrochloric acid needed for digestion, helps distribute hormones, and is necessary to joint and tendon health. Chlorine is found in seaweed, kelp, avocado, tomato, cabbage, kale, turnips, celery, cucumber, asparagus, pineapple, oats, salt, and saltwater fish.

Fluorine and Sexuality

Fluorine strengthens tooth enamel but too much is *not* helpful, as it mottles the teeth. Large amounts of fluorine may also weaken bones and injure internal organs. Sources of fluorine are steel ground oats, sunflower seeds, milk, cheese, carrots, garlic, beet tops, almonds, and green vegetables. You'll have to rely on food sources for both fluorine and chlorine, since neither of these minerals is supplied in multivitamins or in mineral pills.

If nothing else, the foregoing information should bring it home to you and those you love that you are a very complicated piece of machinery and you cannot expect to run efficiently on Cokes, burgers, hot dogs, fries, and ice-cream cones. If your body is poorly supplied, it will not function satisfactorily for your own—or your lover's—sex life. Hopefully, you will take this information to heart as food for thought. And remember that good food and health are the most reliable aphrodisiacs.

Protein and Sexuality

You are mostly made up of protein. Muscles, skin, hair, nails, eyes, heart, blood, lungs, brain, organs, glands, nerves—all are protein. All basic proteins come from animals and plants, *and since you cannot store protein, you need a continuous supply.* You are a twenty-four-hour-a-day repair shop, with some part of your body being overhauled every second. Most of the time you also need energy, so you take what you need and turn it into fuel. Now, here is the catch. To be used for energy, your protein must first be converted into starch or sugar, but once this conversion has taken place, it cannot be changed back. Each and every cell is replaced twice a year, and your liver regenerates every two weeks. If you are under any kind of stress, whether it be getting into a ring with an antagonist or into bed with a protagonist, you need plenty of protein. If you should become ill, you will need even more. As much as 135 grams of first-grade protein can be destroyed in one day fighting illness. Can you imagine the sad plight of a body stricken by illness or accident that has no usable supplies of protein on hand? Can you imagine your own plight if that stricken person happened to be your love?

When you were in school and they talked about hemoglobin, you learned that it picked up oxygen and distributed it to the tissues, where it then picked up carbon dioxide and other wastes for disposal. The fact was not fascinating. But suppose you think of it this way and in connection with your sexuality. What was the effect of poor and inadequate fuel supplies on your life in the last months? What would be the effect on your neighborhood if that lack of fuel prevented garbage collection? In the first instance, things slowed almost to a standstill, and if the second had taken place, there would be a pile-up of filth with every chance of disease. If you don't have an adequate supply of fuel to get you through the day, there is going to be very little energy left for lovemaking or even wanting to make love. If wastes are not disposed of, they poison the system. Oh, not so that you are doubled up and rolling around, but you may well have vague symptoms—aches and pains, bad breath, and body odor—none of which contribute to a happy sex life.

There is another department in your body that is also dependent on good protein; it's rather like a police department and is called gamma globulin. It has its beat in your bloodstream. The force is made up of antibodies which neutralize such bandits as bacteria, viruses, and other unwelcome microorganisms. If you think it has nothing to do with sex, try imagining making love with someone who has a strep throat!

What you did not learn in school is that, while the body of a newborn will follow its built-in instructions step by intricate step to produce energy, the energy can only be as good as the material on hand. It still isn't possible to make gold out of lead, nor can you make high-quality energy from grinders and beer or martinis on the rocks. If even one link in the long chain of changes that occur between putting food in your mouth and having the energy to chew it is weak, the whole apparatus (you) suffers. Ah, you say, but I'm no athlete, I don't need all that much energy, even in bed. Oh, yes you do. Two other vital parts of you, your nervous system and your brain, are dependent on that fuel you are supplying. Your brain may not be athletic, but it is very active and it uses one-quarter of all the glucose carried by your bloodstream. Glucose is the name of your fuel, and it is the only fuel your body can burn. Your essential sugar level (glucose) is maintained directly by your supply of carbohydrates (starches and sugars) and protein. Indirectly, the blood-sugar level is influenced by the amount of fat being burned in your tissues. Hopefully, understanding these little facts is going to change your breakfast habits forever.

Recently "The Inquiring Fotographer" had a column in a metropolitan newspaper. The question he asked was, "Traditionally, Americans have eaten three square meals a day. How many square meals a day do you eat?" The following are the answers from six people who, like you, must get through each day with as much ease and efficiency as possible if they want lovemaking at night. How well do you suppose each of these people might do, and how sexually attractive would you say they were?

Secretary (female). "Only dinner. I skip breakfast completely and I have a very light lunch if I eat at all. I'm conscious of my weight. Sure I'm hungry when I get home at night, but then I eat a meal that is so filling I don't have to snack afterward."

Cashier (male). "Most of us have sedentary jobs, I eat one meal a day and no breakfast at all."

Bank employee (female). "Two square meals, big ones, breakfast is just a coffee break for me. I weigh 170, if I ate three meals a day I'd probably top 200."

Clerk (male). "If you mean by a square meal a sit-down meal, I only have one, in the evening. Breakfast is just coffee. Lunch is pizza and Coke. I wouldn't have time for more anyway, I only get one-half hour for lunch."

Secretary (female). "All I have is one square meal a day. I don't have time for breakfast, and I take my lunch with me so I can sit in the sun."

Section head, brokerage firm (male). "There isn't time for breakfast. My wife works, and I'm not about to give up fifteen minutes of sleep to make myself breakfast. For lunch I have a hot dog or a hamburger. If I get hungry before dinner, I have a bag of potato chips."

Now, let's see what kind of days these people limp through in the light of what they are *not* providing themselves.

All the carbohydrates you eat are transformed into

glucose (sugar), but there is no way of storing that glucose for a later time when you might need it. The very best you could manage in glucose storage would be enough to last you about four to six hours, and most of the energy required by your body during those hours would be right there, traveling around in your bloodstream. Even without a lot of explanation you can see why allowing more than six hours to elapse without taking on additional fuel supplies would put a strain somewhere. During the night, of course, you don't need as much energy as during the day, and it's quite all right to let a couple of extra hours slip past the six-hour deadline. But what about the bodies of those six people? How long do you suppose they go? The first secretary goes twenty-three hours without eating. Can you imagine the number of mistakes her half-starved brain causes her to make? All of the others go seventeen hours without eating anything at all. The one who takes her lunch to work so she can sit in the sun has at least one advantage, possibly three. She *sits* while she eats her lunch, rather than stand up at a lunch counter with the blood pooling in her legs instead of at its appointed place in her stomach. If she brings a really nutritious lunch, that is her second advantage. If it is quiet where she sits, that is the third.

Two of the others go seventeen hours too and then take on a load of very inferior protein in the form of hot dogs, hamburgers, and pizza. The bank employee who goes seventeen hours and then sits down to a big lunch and then five hours later has a big dinner is pretty big herself—but not because she has two meals. One has to ask what it is she orders and how big the portions are. The male cashier who also allows twenty-three hours to elapse between meals couldn't be doing much of a job with his hungry brain either. If his brain uses one-quarter of the glucose available, it's a good thing he doesn't have to add in his head. It is probable that he isn't a giant in bed either.

While *all* of the carbohydrates are transformed into

glucose and none of it can be stored, the story is different for protein. Only half of the protein we eat is transformed into glucose, and it is digested at a much slower rate. That is why, after eating a goodly supply of proteins (bacon and eggs), you don't feel empty at eleven. You aren't. Had your breakfast been the quicker-digested carbohydrates, cereal, toast, or pancakes, your stomach would have begun by then to growl its protest.

Some of your breakfast protein is transformed into glycogen, a form of glucose that can be stored in the liver. That glycogen is available between meals whenever there is a call for energy. However, if you fail to provide your body with protein at breakfast, your blood-sugar level drops within a couple of hours. If you have no stored glycogen to take up the slack, you feel tired, hungry, and cranky. Do any of your co-workers fit that picture?

There is another problem stemming from American breakfast habits, and it is caused by sugar. If you drink a glass of orange juice, you ingest sugar. If you have jam, jelly, marmalade, or honey on your toast, you ingest sugar. If you have syrup on your pancakes, sugar in your coffee, icing on your coffee cake, or even just coffee cake, you ingest sugar. You are, in effect, loaded for bear. Now, your system has been programmed to take certain action under certain conditions, and sugar is one thing that activates an alarm. A message is sent winging to your pancreas that the bloodstream is overloaded with the stuff and orders out the insulin. The pancreas reacts to the frantic call with a large belt of insulin, enough to take care of the overload, and your blood-sugar level drops precipitously. You feel a "sinker" coming on. That's just about the time the refreshment wagon comes around and you purchase a Danish with your coffee—either that or you drop a quarter in the candy machine or pick up a well-sugared Coke. Up shoots your sugar level and you feel human again. A second message has gone out over the wires, however, and the pancreas hits the panic button again.

By the time your lunch hour comes around you are in another "sinker." Whether you handle the problem with a malted or a martini, the effect is the same, and up you go again. By this time, you have established a pattern of peaks and hollows and you couldn't correct it even if you knew what you were doing. There will be another candy bar midafternoon, something on the way home, and a bag of potato chips and a couple of drinks before dinner. How do you think a body on that kind of roller coaster is going to perform in bed? *You* may want to, *it* may not. I wonder if Masters and Johnson ever took the trouble to ask their troubled patients what sort of food habits they had.

There are, of course, people who wouldn't touch a carbohydrate with a nine-foot fork. They are usually the ones on a self-imposed "high-protein diet." As you will see toward the end of this chapter, such diets do encourage weight loss, but there is a catch. Proteins and carbohydrates interact together to maintain the blood-sugar level. If there is an insufficiency of either, then neither can do its best work. The secret of success is not based on either or neither, but on the same principle used in the manufacture of a Rolls-Royce: use the best quality and in the right proportions. There are some surprises for you a few pages on, but at least you won't ever be lost in a wilderness of "latest diets." Nor should you ever again be the victim of food manufacturers and processors who care as much about your sex life as they do about your life—not at all.

Which Protein and How Much?

When any protein is broken down into amino acids, the chemical units that make up protein, it is they and not the price, grade, or taste that determine the biological and nutritive value. It is nice, in this time (which will last a long time) of high-priced beef, to know that hamburger has exactly the same protein value as sirloin steak. To use amino acids to best advantage, you have to use the right assortment. The best way to explain amino acids, which I'm sure you tuned out in school, is by way of football, which I am equally sure you kept tuned into.

As in football, in which there must be twenty-two men on the field if a game is to take place, there are twenty-two amino acids. Eight of these are called essential, not because they are any more important than the others; they are all equally important. The essential ones have that tag attached because they live outside the city limits, so to speak, while the other fourteen not only live in town, they live right there on the stadium grounds. Fourteen amino acids can be produced right there in your body and are ready to play at any time. The other eight, which are termed essential, like the eight commuting football players who come in by bus, must be brought in from other sources via the food you select for your diet.

Once you understand that all twenty-two players, including the bus riders, are absolutely necessary for the game (protein synthesis), then, like any good coach, you ought to consider the strengths that each individual player brings with him. The essential eight are the key, because while you have control over the fourteen living in, those eight boys in the bus are another story. If seven are in great shape but the eighth, who happens to be your prize passer, suffers a shoulder separation while riding his bike to the movies, the game isn't going to get into the air. Even if the shoulder isn't a total disaster and your eighth player actually gets into the game, he isn't going to be very effective. If for best results the team needs *all* of those eight in 100-percent condition and one can only deliver 50 percent, then the final score is going to reflect the weakest member.

If the protein you eat delivers those eight essential amino acids in the right proportion, then you will derive 100-percent value from the action. If seven arrive with 100 percent, but one brings in only 50 percent, then you might just as well have taken in only 50 percent of the other seven.

Your body can only use one pattern of essential amino acids, and the biological value of any protein is determined by how nearly it fits that pattern. In other words, that pattern represents the percentage of absorbed protein your body actually uses. This is called NPU, Net Protein Utilization, and is analogous to the amount of firepower we can expect from those eight guys on the bus. Just as it would be helpful to know what each man can contribute to the game, knowing what each food can contribute to your actual needs would be helpful. Of what value would it be to eat constantly of only the tastiest, most expensive, perfectly prepared protein if the body can only use a small percentage of that particular protein we have selected?

The protein that best matches the body's utilization pattern is the one found in eggs—and before we go any further, we should discuss eggs.

What Is Actually Known About Eggs?

They are the most nearly perfect, naturally occurring protein food we have. Egg protein is the yardstick against which all other proteins are measured because it fits the needs of the human body.

The essential amino acids are all found in eggs.

The protein-to-fat ratio in eggs is the highest of that in any easily available food.

The high iron content of eggs is of excellent quality and is already combined with the protein, so it is in a biologically available form.

Eggs are rich in thiamine, riboflavin, and vitamins A and D.

Eggs are *not* high in saturated fats, said to play a part in atherosclerosis.

There is no indication that the consumption of eggs, even in large quantities, will increase the risk of heart attack.

Many doctors and researchers believe that the high quality of the protein in eggs is needed by heart patients when rebuilding the damaged heart muscle.

A group of men and a doctor, Walter G. Goodale, of Boston's Peter Bent Brigham Hospital, went on a diet which included twenty-four eggs a day every day for several weeks. The serum cholesterol level dropped in every man, and because they were on a low-calorie diet, they all lost weight.

In the Ireland-Boston Heart Study, researchers followed six hundred Irishmen between the ages of thirty and sixty who had lived in Boston for ten years or more, and their brothers, who had never left the old country. The Irish brothers ate about twice as many eggs as the American brothers (averaging well over fourteen a week), yet the Irish brothers had lower levels of cholesterol in their bloodstreams. In the category of disease, their hearts were rated from two to six times as healthy as the Boston brothers'. It is assumed that *stress* accounted for the difference.

Dr. Michael DeBakey, one of the world's leading heart surgeons, and his research team studied 1,700 patients hospitalized for the surgical treatment of severe cases of atherosclerosis. Eight out of ten of those patients had cholesterol levels within the *normal* range for Americans.

Dr. Harold Kahn of the National Heart and Lung Institute has reported that despite the widely publicized hypothesis that dietary cholesterol causes heart attacks, there has been virtually no change in the proportion of cholesterol consumed over the past sixty years. During that same period, however, the heart-attack rate has skyrocketed.

Those are the things that are *known* about eggs, and it isn't guesswork. Furthermore, we also know that heart attacks were almost unknown in the days when eggs were the reason every farm had a hen house. We also know that eggs contain all of the essential amino acids—no guesswork there either.

Here are a few facts which may help you pick and choose intelligently at the supermarket whose owners would really rather you didn't.

1. There are many sources of protein that rank higher than meat. Soybean flour is an example.
2. Cheeses too are high.
3. Meat is not much higher than lentils, which cost much less.
4. Eggs and milk are higher than meat.
5. Soybeans and *whole* rice are at the top.
6. Meat's advantage is that we need less of it to fulfill our needs.
7. Plant protein's advantage is that it contains fewer calories.
8. *All* meats are high in Net Protein Utilization, and it makes no difference which ones you serve.

So, to round off your lesson in basic nutrition which your teachers should have made intelligible long ago so that you could have protected your health, sexuality, and your heart, you need to know about enzymes. Back to the football field.

Enzymes are like the football itself. They promote action but are not themselves used up in that action. The football gets everybody going, but after the play is completed there sits the football on the ground, just about the same as it was before.

In your body there are many, many enzymes, each acting on a very limited set of chemical reactions, but virtually nothing goes on within you without the direction of one enzyme or another. If your diet is adequate, then your system can produce a number of its own enzymes, and every time you ingest live, raw food, you take on more. A sure way to help the enzymes you have working for you is to finish off your meal with a slice of apple, papaya, or pineapple, as these fruits contain the most enzymes of any fruits and will help to break down both proteins and fats. The enzyme ptyalin in your mouth goes to work on any carbohydrate that passes that way, provided you don't gulp!

You need a constant supply of enzymes, and they are found *only* in fresh, wholesome foods. Processing destroys them, so always ask yourself, as you wander up and down the aisles at the supermarket, where colorful treasures beckon from every shelf: Has it been processed? If yes, be selective. You may feed your *mouth* with a few of them. After all, you were programmed at a very early age to believe what the advertisements said, and at a very early age your perfectly good taste buds were corrupted (like mine) in favor of some very processed foods indeed. But use your brain as you choose from the perhaps limited but still very worthwhile foods that will feed your whole body and your brain. In the next section, on diets, you will see that while the supermarket is a vast city of shelves, those in your house are limited and the number of calories you may consume each and every day is also limited. If you load those shelves with processed, nutritionally dead, but highly caloric foods, there will be little room for other things. In the end you will be fat, sluggish, flabby, sallow, tired—and about as sexy as a mop.

Diet

To diet or not to diet? is not a question too many Americans have to ask themselves. Men or women, girls or boys, rich or poor—millions of them simply must diet. The reason is not surplus food but rather the type of foods they eat, the amount of food they eat, *the time of day they eat it*, the stresses under which they live, and their sedentary habits. If you find that you are overweight (check with weights and measurements), there is virtually no way to lose that weight by diet alone; you will have to add some form of exercise to your life. By the same token, an increase in exercise plus an increase in food intake, while making you stronger, won't slim you. It is going to take a combination of both, but there are ways to cut down on calories, lose weight, and feel absolutely fine, even if you eat from stress. But first you will need some protective information about diets.

Diet does not necessarily mean eating less. It is merely a word connected with what is eaten. The latest leaning in America today seems to be the low carbohydrate diet. It took quite a long time to get here from England, where it was invented in 1862 by a Dr. William Harvey, Fellow of the Royal College of Surgeons, Aural Surgeon to the Great Northern Hospital, Surgeon to the Royal Dispensary of the Ear, and not at all the type of fellow who might be considered a faddist. Dr. Harvey felt that since sugar and starch were used to fatten animals, it was quite possible that they might also fatten people. He was also concerned with diabetes, and since sugar had something to do with diabetes, perhaps diabetes might return the favor and have something to do with obesity. In any event, he decided that a "diet" made up of animal flesh plus vegetables having little sugar or starch might be helpful. He designed a diet for one of his portly patients, one Mr. Banting. It added up to 3,000 calories a day, and of those 3,000 calories *sixty grams* were composed of carbohydrates. You will note that the good doctor took note of Mr. Banting's fondness for the "cup," which was as customary in 1862 as today. He did suggest that Mr. Banting take some exercise, but there is no record that this part of his advice was followed. Should you wish to try the diet, you can be assured at the outset: it works.

Breakfast

4 to 8 ounces of meat (four would be an average serving in a good restaurant today)

2 ounces biscuits or toast (that would be one and a half whole-wheat muffins—the *real* whole wheat kind)

A large cup of tea or coffee, no sugar or milk

Dinner (at midday)

10 to 12 ounces of any fish except salmon

Any vegetable except potatoes or other root vegetables
A slice of poultry or venison (beef would do as well now that it's no longer corn-fed)
2 ounces of toasted bread
2 to 3 glasses of good red wine, sherry, or Madeira—no champagne, port, or beer.

Afternoons
4 to 6 ounces of fruit
1 or 2 biscuits

Supper
6 to 8 ounces of meat or fish
1 or 2 glasses of red wine
Bread—if too dry, moisten with brandy

On that sumptuous, but carefully selected fare, Mr. Banting lost fifty pounds in one year, and everybody who was anybody went "A-banting." The medical society of the day reacted much as our own do today; they almost did Dr. Harvey in.

The Ice Cap Diet

Thirty-four years later an explorer by the name of Vihjalmar Stefansson added weight to Harvey's discovery quite by accident. As thoroughly addicted to sugar and carbohydrates as the next man, he was suddenly separated from them when the polar ice moved in ahead of the party he was supposed to join and he had to spend the winter with a group of Eskimos. Their diet consisted of seal blubber, bear, raw fish, and caribou. It wasn't the sort of diet the average person would choose, but fortunately there was no choice. As the weeks passed, Stefansson noticed that his physical condition was improving markedly and he began paying intelligent attention to the incredible health and good looks of his hosts, coming to the conclusion that food must play a key role.

On Stefansson's return to civilization he tried to interest others in his discovery and met with the usual frustrations, but he was a tenacious man and, still trying twenty-two years later, he decided that only a radical experiment would prove his theories. Under the watchful eyes of several doctors he began a three-month stay at New York City's Bellevue Hospital living on nothing but fat meat and water. On 3,000 calories a day he lost ten pounds in that time (about the same as Banting) and lowered his blood-serum cholesterol. He was in topnotch condition and the so-called "well-balanced diet" began to lose some of its aura. He didn't spend the rest of his life on fat meat and water, but he did limit his intake of carbohydrates.

Sixteen years later a longtime friend of Stefansson, Dr. Blake Donaldson, put his overweight patients at the New York Hospital on a low-carbohydrate, high-fat diet. The experiment was a success, but the medical establishment was still quite "sot" in its ways.

Coming a little closer to today was an experiment ordered by the Du Pont Company. Dr. Alfred Pennington, who was working in their Medical Research Department, was asked to devise something that would help the company's overweight employees. On his program the executives and their wives in the study also ate up to 3,000 calories a day and the average weight loss was twenty-two pounds in three and a half months. That was even a little better than Banting, but you'll see why in a minute.

At each and every meal

½ pound of meat with its fat (one part fat to three parts meat)

One portion of *one* of the foods on the following list—*no* seconds.

White or sweet potato

Boiled rice

Grapefruit, grapes, melon, bananas, pears, blueberries, or raspberries

Black coffee or tea

I tried it and used the list to make the following combinations and found that they worked well.

Breakfast
Melon, broiled steak, and tea

Lunch
Broiled chicken with rice, coffee

Dinner
Baked fish and sweet potatoes

The reason for my particular selections were simple. I *longed* for rice and potatoes. I dearly loved melon. Grapefruit, grapes, bananas, and berries aren't all that important to me. I didn't object to the repetitions, and as the pounds melted away, I objected even less.

The Tale of Taller

In 1953 the *New England Journal of Medicine* published Dr. Pennington's paper, *Reorientation on Obesity.* He too set a limit of sixty grams for carbohydrates, and while the average citizen did not have access to the article, presumably Dr. Taller did. He changed things around a little and came out with a book called *Calories Don't Count*. Most of us thought it was pretty silly; how could we be expected to follow all that stuff, along with three ounces of safflower oil. Safflower oil was Dr. Taller's gimmick, and it had to be safflower oil. Education in school and at home had always indicated that oil was fat, fat was fat, and you should stay away from it.

There probably wasn't much wrong with the Taller presentation of an idea that should have been aired years ago, but there *was* something wrong with the title of his book. Calories *do* count, it's just that some count less than others. Dr. Taller went into "business" with some people who had far less to lose than he, and they formed a corporation to sell safflower-oil capsules, which the good doctor advertised in his book. It was understood that two of the magic capsules taken before each meal would do the three-ounce safflower job. Advertising a brand-name drug or product in a book is illegal, and that was his punishable mistake. He did, however, make another. Two capsules taken three times a day add up to six. On investigation it was later shown that it would take eighty-four capsules a day to make up the three ounces of safflower the doctor had prescribed. A slight miscalculation of seventy-eight capsules.

And Along Came Stillman

Dr. Irwin Stillman carried the low-carbohydrate diet one step further into the *no-carbohydrate* class. He adhered to the current medically accepted idea that fat makes fat and it is therefore to be avoided. If you recall, we said earlier that carbohydrates interact with proteins and that if one is totally absent the other cannot do its best work. Dr. Stillman overlooked this fact of nutrition.

One of the results of carbohydrate deprivation is called "ketosis," which has for its symptoms bad breath, throat dryness, nausea, irritability, and excess acid in both blood and urine. While it is true that weight loss does occur with the Stillman "Water Diet," people can stay on it for only limited periods. When they return to their normal eating patterns, the weight returns. It is not a sensible way to eat or to live, and until both can be handled sensibly, obesity cannot be controlled.

Enter Dr. Atkins

Dr. Robert C. Atkins knew what Dr. Taller knew, and that is: Gimmicks sell things. And he has an interesting one; it's called a *keto stick*. He too uses the idea of carbohydrate limitation, and like Stillman, recommends cutting out *all* carbohydrates at the start. He differs, however, in two important areas. One, he does not go along with the medical establishment, which says fat is fat, cut it out. Stefansson, in an effort to prove that fat played a highly beneficial role in nutrition, *particularly in the absence of carbohydrates,* confined himself, for a period while he was in the dietetic ward at Bellevue, to a diet of just lean meat. He soon felt its effects (as he had at one time when in the arctic and was deprived of fat) and developed diarrhea, fatigue, and a flock of other unpleasant symptoms. He then "cured" himself by adding fat to his diet. Atkins' second important difference is that while he *starts* his dieters off on a diet devoid of carbohydrates, it is for a limited period only. He suggests one week as a good start, and this is where the gimmick comes in. The dieter can test his urine daily with a keto stick (available in drugstores), and if the diet is working the keto stick will turn purple and it is then implied that you are on the road to a slimmer figure. Actually, when the stick turns purple you are in that state of ketosis mentioned earlier. In that state Dr. Atkins says you are forced to call on your stored fat, which then slowly melts away. After a week of total abstention from *any* carbohydrates, the keto stick should certainly provide the cheering news (some people hold out for two) that a slim figure is indeed on the way. Then Dr. Atkins suggests five grams of carbohydrate be ingested daily for a week and then an additional five grams on the second week, bringing the total to ten. This goes on with a weekly increase of five grams until the grand total of forty is reached. This was the same number as that suggested by Dr. Pennington to patients who couldn't lose on sixty grams.

The trouble with *Dr. Atkins' Diet Revolution* is really the American people. Have you ever noticed how they feel about medicine? Have you ever heard of anyone asking for or being offered *one* aspirin? Probably not. Our whole philosophy is, if one is good, two are better. Many who went on the Atkins diet found that they did lose weight and, as promised, they "turned purple." That is to say their urine turned the keto sticks purple, a sure sign, according to Dr. Atkins, that the "fat mobilizing hormone" was at work. With delight they accepted the new diet, which not only satisfied their hunger, but really worked, even without a speck of carbohydrate. Once they started to lose weight and turn purple, they just decided to keep her a-goin'. For many this just couldn't work out, and they began to experience mild symptoms of ketosis, bad breath, and some fatigue. Some went completely out of whack, suffered from diarrhea, lost valuable nutrients because of it, swelled up, and gave the medical establishment just the ammunition they needed to shoot down yet another low-carbohydrate diet.

One of Dr. Atkins' critics wrote, "The Atkins diet is nonsense. Coronary heart disease is the principal cause of death in the United States, and any diet that tends to be high in saturated fats and cholesterol tends to elevate the chance that the individual will get heart disease. Any book that recommends unlimited amounts of meat, butter, and eggs, as this one does, is in my opinion dangerous. The author who makes the suggestion is guilty of malpractice."

The only diet I know of that goes in for the word "unlimited" is the one erroneously called "the Mayo diet," which suggests two eggs and two slices of bacon as a minimum, and you may have as much as twelve eggs and twelve slices of bacon if you wish. At both luncheon and dinner you are offered all the meat and salad you can eat, and even gravy in any amount, provided it does not contain sugar or flour. The Mayo Clinic disowns this diet, and so does anyone who tries it overlong. There is no such thing as "all you want."

The critic of the Atkins diet was correct in one statement only: coronary disease is the principal cause of death in the United States. As far as meat and fats and cholesterol are concerned, keep in mind the year that Stefansson ate nothing but fat meat and water. He lost weight and *significantly lowered his cholesterol level.* The same thing happened to men who ate nothing but eggs for several weeks at Peter Bent Brigham. The two villains who have no such studies to prove their innocence are refused admittance to the Atkins diet; they are flour and sugar.

But meat is expensive, even though you like it very much. The person who is used to crisp salads or who raises delicious vegetables in summer, freezing and canning them also for winter use, will soon long for variety. What we really need to know is which proteins have value and yet are not too expensive in terms of calories, which *do* count. We already know that we need a certain number of grams of carbohydrate, but how many? Thirty is listed as the minimum and sixty as the maximum, but those numbers didn't come off the ten commandments—they are meant as guideposts. If your diet keeps you satisfied at sixty grams a day and you don't need to lose, great, you have hit on the magic number. If you do need to lose, you will have to consume fewer grams of carbohydrate. But just which ones do you cut out?

It has occurred to many people that some foods have fewer carbohydrate grams than others, just as some foods, whether protein, fat, or carbohydrate, have fewer calories. If one could make two lists, one enumerating foods by their caloric content and the other by their carbohydrate gram content, it would be no trick at all to see how to diet with the most in food variety and the least in calories and grams. After trying to concoct different lists on my own, I found that Donald S. Mart had already figured one out most scientifically in his book *The Carbo-Calorie Diet*. He measures a food's caloric and carbohydrate gram content by what he calls the *carbo-calorie*. Mr. Mart says you can't actually combine a calorie with a gram of carbohydrate except as a means of mathematical measurement. But if such a mathematical combination works and is really helpful (and it is), then I say, for the first time in my life: Hurrah for Math!

You will find the carbo-calorie count for most foods

in Mr. Mart's book and it's therefore a very handy book to have. You will also find the formula for determing a carbo-calorie for any strange and exotic foods not listed in his book. But that's not the way I used it. I listed all the foods that cost *one* carbo-calorie (you are permitted no more than 100 a day, and only 75 if you wish to lose weight). I then listed all the twos and so on. It was an education in itself. I found for instance that *one* pecan equaled one large egg. There is no contest there. The egg has all of the amino acids and also quiets hunger pangs. That pecan is also equal to one spear of asparagus or one-half cup of chard leaves (the stems are more expensive). When I moved on to two carbo-calories, I could choose between six slices of cucumber or one lichee nut. I could have one-half cup of boiled cabbage, one animal cracker, or two lettuce leaves for the same two carbo-calories.

Jumping to four, I found lots of good vegetables which, alas, were always measured by the half cup—and if you like vegetables you know you'll probably eat enough to cost you eight carbo-calories. Most liquor in the amount of 1½ ounces also costs four, but you may only have one chocolate kiss for the same price.

Cheeses abound in the five-carbo-calorie department, as do fish (four ounces), chicken, beef, and wine—which now clears up the amounts allowed Mr. Banting. Five will also buy you one-half cup of puffed rice.

Six is strong on organ meats and also includes many soups (one-half cup, which means a decent serving costs twelve). For six you may also have one marshmallow or one Lorna Doone or one Uneeda Biscuit!

Seven will buy the more exotic seafoods, such as lobster salad, shrimp, mussels, and tuna. You can also have one-half cup of chard leaves *and* their stalks. One-half cup of buttermilk is listed right next to one-half cup of cottage cheese. (I used to drink a quart of the one and eat a whole container of the other and think I was dieting.) Most cocktails cost seven.

You have to reach eight before fruit appears. Both

skim and whole milk are in this range, as is *one* caramel or *one* Toll House cookie.

We had to wait until nine before candy showed up in force, if you can call *one* bon bon, *one* gum drop, *one* sour ball or *one* piece of butterscotch "in force." Liqueurs (one ounce) cost nine, and so does *one* Rye Krisp. I guess you thought you were dieting too!

Ten ushers in stew, cole slaw, and one pancake.

Eleven sees the first piece of cake, a square of devil's food. Of course, you might prefer one-half cup of ready-to-eat-oatmeal.

Twelve is what lots of folks have been waiting for, bread and cereals. You can have one piece of rye, whole-wheat, or cracked-wheat bread, or one-half cup of Krispies, Pep, Post Toasties, Rice Krispies, Wheat Flakes or Wheaties—but don't forget to add the carbo-calories for milk, sugar, butter, jam, jelly, marmalade, honey, and fruit. For twelve you might prefer a fig bar or one-half cup of grapefruit or orange juice.

You have to pay thirteen for one-half cup of lemonade or unsweetened applesauce.

Fourteen brings on all the old winter standbys: Cream of Wheat, Farina, Maypo, Oatmeal . . . and the first sugared cereal, Sugar Krisps. Soft drinks come under fourteen (measured as four ounces, when everybody knows there's no such thing as a half-glass or half-bottle of soda). However, you can have a beer for fourteen, all eight ounces.

Four ounces of bacon comes in at fifteen (yes, you are going to need a little scale) and so does *one* Parker House roll. You can have *one* chocolate-covered cherry or one-half pink grapefruit or one-half cup of chocolate milk, or one manhattan. Remember, most other cocktails cost seven and that means two martinis to one manhattan!

One ear of corn will cost sixteen, or you could have a slice of pumpernickel, one brownie, or one-half cup of Grapenuts. For the same price you could have a two-egg Spanish omelet.

One-half cup of bananas goes for seventeen, and so does one-half cup of corn, custard, tapioca, or vanilla pudding. If you are a cookie buff, you may have *one* Oreo. The grown-ups can have a Tom Collins.

For eighteen you may have *one* cheese blintze (I've written "blintze" in the singular, but it's usually consumed in the plural), a banana fritter, one-half cup of Jell-O, or one fresh apple. Alas, how ignorant we were!

Nineteen ushers in fish and scallops fried in batter, or you might prefer one-half cup of chili con carne (double one-half cup, or 38 carbo-calories, sounds more realistic). Wheatena costs nineteen, and so does one *plain* doughnut. Mark that down; worse is to follow. You may have only one tablespoon of fudge or butterscotch sauce.

For twenty carbo-calories you may have one baking-powder biscuit or one-half cup of either noodles or macaroni, or four ounces of potato salad. You can have one rye-'n'-ginger.

For twenty-one you may have one Shredded Wheat biscuit. If you are the mother of a baby you should be aware that there are twenty-one carbo-calories in one ounce of infants' dry precooked cereal. For twenty-one you may have one-half cup of peas, limas, or corn, one medium baked potato, one whole-wheat roll, one frankfurter roll (without the frank), one piece of gold cake, eight ounces of potato soup, or an eight-ounce can of beef stew.

One chocolate cream costs twenty-two and so does a hamburger roll. (See why you should order Salisbury steak instead?) You could choose to have a French roll, four ounces of cooked white rice or puffed oats, a chocolate éclair, or one glass of gingerale.

Twenty-three gives you a wonderful example of choices. You may have one-half of a fryer chicken, one-half cup of corned-beef hash, four ounces of salami, one cupcake, or one pretzel!

It was with real sorrow that I discovered that one-half cup of pork and beans would cost me twenty-four. I would shoot my whole daily allotment of seventy-five right there, if I ventured so much as one bite. For twenty-four I could have one slice of pound cake, a cruller, one-half cup of Wheat Chex, a Coke, or a root beer.

For twenty-five you can have one piece of cornbread, an avocado, one-half cup of mashed banana (mothers of young babies beware), or a cup of Rice Flakes.

By the time we reach twenty-six, most of the nutritious foods have been covered and the list runs off into muffins, buns, stuffing, and cake. You could have one-half cup of macaroni salad or four ounces of fruit salad . . . and I used to think I was both Spartan and calorically frugal when I ate fruit salad.

Twenty-seven carbo-calories are found in fruit cocktail with fruit syrup or French toast with maple syrup. It is under twenty-seven that we find our first sandwich, lettuce and tomato, and also a gin and tonic.

If you feel like having three gumdrops, it will cost you twenty-eight, and so will a medium lollipop, the kind children are given in the doctor's office. However, if you are hungry you may have a sliced chicken or tuna sandwich. You can quench your thirst with a grape or lemon soda. For dessert, you may select a doughnut, iced this time, or yogurt with fruit. Surprised?

If you had a cheese omelet with two slices of bacon, it would cost you only sixteen. But one Danish or one raisin muffin is going to cost you twenty-nine.

For thirty you could have a ham, tongue, or roast-beef sandwich, but it would be wiser to have a whole pound of turkey. One large hard roll will also cost thirty, but its value in nutrition is nowhere near its value in carbo-calories.

At thirty-one a large number of cakes appear on the list, and we see the first sign of a pizza. A half-pint of vanilla ice cream also falls in this range, but any one of these foods nudges a dieter's carbo-calorie intake up to almost half his daily dose.

One bagel costs thirty-two. Couldn't you settle for lox

and cream cheese? They have good nutritional value and cost only sixteen. You could even throw in some sliced onion for next to nothing.

Thirty-three—french pastry.

Thirty-four—hamburgers and cheeseburgers.

Thirty-five—chocolate pudding, one-half cup of french fries, or a jelly doughnut.

Thirty-six—baked apple with two tablespoons of sugar, one and one-half cup of Wheat Chex, chocolate chiffon pie, or one piece of almond coffee cake.

Thirty-seven—bacon-lettuce-and-tomato sandwich, a peanut-butter sandwich, one-half pint of strawberry ice cream, or one slice of iced coffee cake with nuts.

Thirty-eight—coffee ice cream or one-half cup of spaghetti with meat sauce.

Thirty-nine—one square of plain butter cake.

Forty-one—one tablespoon of caramel sauce.

Forty-two—banana cream pie.

Forty-five—all ice-cream sodas.

Fifty—devil's food cake, iced.

Fifty-three—chicken TV dinner.

Fifty-four—frozen beef pot pie.

Fifty-seven—cream-cheese-and-jelly sandwich.

Fifty-nine—one piece of chocolate layer cake.

Sixty-two—strawberry cream pie.

Sixty-three—hot fudge sundae.

Sixty-four—strawberry shortcake.

One hundred—banana split.

You would be very wise to use a cut-off line. After twenty-five, the nutritional value goes down, as the carbo-calorie count goes up. There is only one way to hold yourself to a cut-off line: keep the foods above your cut-off line out of the house. Don't make your dietary lapses easy to fall into by keeping pizza in the freezer and cookies in the cupboard. Make it harder than that—and more rewarding—by making cookies and pizza a treat rather than a habit. Get out of the house and drive, bike, or walk to get those occasional treats. That way you're less likely to eat junk food on a whim, and your round-trip bike or walk may even burn up those extra carbo-calories you indulge in.

Keep your proteins coming at a regular pace; in other words, don't skip meals. I always keep a bowl of hard-boiled eggs in the refrigerator. You can eat them whole or make marvelous deviled eggs by mixing cottage cheese, mayonnaise, and mustard with the yolks. Hard-boiled eggs can also be sliced or mashed and served with French dressing. I call them emergency rations, and they make all the difference.

Try a sandwich made up of a slice of meat between two slices of cheese; it is high in nutrition and low in calories. Children are big on snacks, but they *don't* need chocolate in their milk and, most of all, they don't need sodas, candy, cookies or ice cream as a regular thing. Try snacking on slim strips of meat such as turkey, ham, or bologna. Keep cheese squares, bacon bits, and crispy fresh vegetables ready at hand.

Do you know why holidays once seemed so wonderfully exciting and why today they seem like commercial commonplaces? It's because life was once so hard, so demanding, and so filled with work that taking time off was like celebrating a holy day; it was a heavenly change. Holidays were special because every day wasn't a holiday. By the same token, ice cream was special because it appeared only on special occasions, a piece of rock candy was something you looked forward to all week, and an ice-cream soda was rare indeed. Those things were scarce in people's lives because they were expensive. They're still expensive today, but the major part of the price you pay is in carbo-calories and health. People in the old days may not have had quite the quantity or variety of food that we do, but they didn't die for lack of nutritious food. We do die because of a lack of understanding and knowledge about nutrition. With the foregoing chapters in mind, look at the people you love; don't just look, *see*. And then remember that what you are, and even how long you are, depends in large part on your diet.

13

Playtime

When I was in high school I had to attend a series of lectures labelled "Sex Ed." They were delivered by a very rotund woman doctor who was long on statistics and, I felt, must be correspondingly short on personal experience. She could, however, be devastatingly frank when asked a question within that experience. One query brought forth an answer so frightening and so laden with truth that while I have forgotten virtually every other answer given me by any other teacher I can remember, I can still recite that one, word for unhappy word. "How often do people make love?" asked my idiot seatmate. She *always* asked idiot questions. Who *cared* how often people made love! The dumpy little doctor looked out at us over the top of her bifocals and smiled sadly, a little as though she wished no one had asked. There we sat, thirty nubile adolescents for whom the very words *make love* were aphrodisiac, attending a class about sex when what we really wanted was to be out in the field sampling it. I wondered why she found the question sad, and then I found out.

"Making love is like getting a new hat," she said. "At first you wear it all the time, and then, as time passes, you wear it less and less." With that awful insight that often makes adolescence a nightmare filled with things you would rather not know, I was thrown into a panic. I was still young enough to hear what people didn't say as well as what they did say, and sometimes even more clearly. What she didn't say was: "and finally the poor old thing gets pushed to the back of the shelf and one day is tossed out along with the one-eyed teddy bear and the busted tin soldier." Suddenly I understood that sad smile and it shook me right down to my saddle shoes. *That lady was sorry for us.* She was sorry for all the hurts we would suffer, and she was sorry that for all our high expectations and resolves, we too would find our fine millinery faded and in two words "old hat." We had four more Sex Ed classes after that one, but I didn't learn anything more. I guess the story of what happens to lovemaking was the only thing I did learn, but it changed my life. Maybe it will change yours.

That the little doctor spoke the truth cannot be questioned. Today's divorce rate backs her up one hundred percent. The remarriage rate bespeaks eloquently of the search for new hats which don't seem to have any greater durability than the discards, but I did find exceptions. There *are* people who seem to keep their excitement and desire for one another bright and shining, and when I was trying to discover if there were things these people had in common, I tried to apply adages from my own limited supply. One, provided me by my mother when she was admonishing me on choosing a husband, warned, "When poverty stalks in by the door, love flies out the window." I could certainly see how poverty's attendants, fear, worry, and deprivation, would sorely try love, but I soon discovered that the security of wealth wasn't able to bar the windows with any greater success. Rich folks threw their old hats away with even greater alacrity than those in less comfortable circumstances. No, it had to be something else. Finally it all boiled down to some very simple things that could almost be considered a syndrome since they were almost always found together. The happy ones were healthy and quite active. They kept a certain childlike quality in their play—*and they set great store by vacations.* They permitted nothing to prevent vacations or to interrupt them, and while the wealthy had longer and more expensive vacations than the less affluent, there the difference ended. What they all had in common can be found in the dictionary next to the word *vacation*. "Vacatio, onis, vacare," to be *empty*, to have *time*, to be *free*. As far as I can see, the Latin "Vacatio, onis, vacare" is just as important to the maintenance of sexuality and happiness as "amo, amat, amamis." In fact, the latter are very dependent upon the former.

There is even something in the Bible about entering the Kingdom of Heaven (which state isn't so very different from loving and being loved) and the necessity to become as little children. If you put all these things together you begin to realize that the secret of maintaining excitement in lovemaking cannot be found in how-to books, nor in new partners. It lies in continual *growth and change*, the kind one finds always in children, occasionally in adults, and almost never in those who toss their old hats out every second or third spring.

New babies are totally intuitive. They know all about the feelings their mothers have, even before they are born. Once they get here, they read everyone who comes near them, and they do so with lines of communication that are all the better for not being jammed by words. Babies are happily *empty* of worries and problems. They have lots of *time* to spend on growing and changing, and they are totally *free* of responsibilities. It's a pity they can't really appreciate it, having nothing as yet with which to compare. But whether or not it is appreciated is of no importance; what is important is that it be used for *growth and change*.

When babies grow into little kids, they lose a lot of their intuition, but since they had so much in the beginning, the loss does not pauperize them. They keep right on reading people, but now against the handicap of the spoken word. Grown-ups are rarely totally honest with children, but then, they aren't really honest with themselves most of the time. Children soon discover that they have to separate what is said from what is felt, which is often confusing but very handy in the game called "Divide and Conquer." In pitting one parent against the other, children are always ahead, they know exactly how far to push and also in which direction for each parent.

When you apply the three principles of *vacatio* to children, you can easily see that they are still in full force. Little kids can *empty* their heads whenever they want to. They lie on their backs and watch cloud camels turn into cloud dragons, and they never once think about the multiplication tables. Or they lie on their fronts watching an ant push a huge beetle up a hill and down a hole. It doesn't remind them even once about the chores they are supposed to be doing. They just watch and dream and *grow and change.*

Kids have *time* too, and they do magical things with it. They are filled with the blessed narcotic of endlessness. For kids there are a billion tomorrows. Best of all, they are still *free,* and what they are free of is responsibility, even for themselves. The full use of *vacatio* in everyday living permits children to be constantly in touch with their own inner selves, a part of each of us that we have named most inadequately *The Unconscious. Other* conscious might be better, for this inner self is highly developed and of the utmost importance. It never sleeps, and it forgets nothing. Little children consult constantly with that part of themselves, and as a result, they *change and grow* at express speeds.

Then they go to school, and deterioration begins. There is less time to be alone and there is less freedom of every kind. Even preschoolers are robbed of about forty hours of self-communion each week by television. It becomes more and more difficult to empty their heads because things begin to have names and limiting descriptions that put a ceiling on dreaming. Descriptions that contribute nothing to the creative art of imagining something out of nothing. *Growth and change* begin to slow down, and if something doesn't come along to interrupt the trend, it will lead eventually to dullness and that lack of inner excitement that brings on the destruction of sexuality. What comes along to save the day is *vacation*—and often, just in time. After those many long months of being penned indoors separated from their inner selves by the intrusions of school (not so very different from your job), the doors open and the children escape. Once again they can *empty* their heads, spend *time* doing what appears to be nothing—and they are *free*. What is the result of this happy combination? *Growth and change.* Surely you can remember saying in September when classes reconvened, "Gee! So-and-so is *changed,* he used to be such a pain, but he's sure *changed.*" It wasn't that So-and-so was merely taller or fatter or faster on the field, he was actually *changed* somewhere inside, and you couldn't say just how or what. In any case, you found him interesting and you had to get to know him all over again. Translated to sexuality, this change would be just as good as a new hat—better, because since the change was self-generated, all the advantages of newness would be present, but there would be no loss of the known and endearing characteristics.

Then we all grow up. Intuition recedes alarmingly as the use of words jams our once-sensitive receivers. There is no longer *time* to watch clouds go by, and every waking moment is filled with *doing*. There is so much stir and noise around us that we can't hear ourselves anymore, and most people get out of the habit of listening. For fifty weeks a year we fight racket, crowds, and problems. *Time* is turned over to the hamburger machine known as schedules, and the wonderful, interesting, informative, and creative inner self is ignored. Instead of *growing and changing* so that we are beings with a thousand hats, we turn dull, and those closest to us know exactly what we are going to say and do—even before we know ourselves. And that is what the story of the discarded hat is all about. Now to the safeguards that can turn aside this dismal fate.

The children who changed so noticeably over their vacations managed to get out of the rut that work and repetition forced them into. *Change* came about when they went back to communing with themselves. This is really what is behind much of the meditation that is going on today. When you meditate you do what you once did so naturally as a child. In other times life was such that even grown-ups had a natural opportunity to commune with themselves as they walked the long miles to and from work or sat quietly under a full moon at day's end. Such opportunities are no longer ours by right, but we do still have the right to a vacation. If you really understand your danger and if you really understand the tremendous value of vacations properly planned for and undertaken, not only will you be able to enhance your sexuality and your life, you will possess an unequaled treasure—a passport to yourself.

The word *vacation* has yet another meaning: *to get away from.* So ask yourself what it is in your life you would like to escape. Sit down and make a list; then apply that list to your vacation plans. Do you want to get away from noise and crowds? Then don't take a room on the Grand Canal in Venice or in the center of *any* city, no matter what cultural advantages they offer. And don't go to Disneyland! Is it people you want to escape? Then leave the tours alone. No tour can guarantee that the people you will be sharing your vacation with are your kind of people, and there's no getting away from them once the plane takes off. Do you want to get out of the kitchen? Then why are you planning to rent a trailer? You'd like to get away from the kids for a while, but with today's prices the only way you can all have a vacation is together and in a trailer? All right, but where are you planning to go? If you investigate ahead of time, you will be able to locate places that cater to all ages and provide plenty of diversion. If the kids are all busy, then there will be time for you to spend on yourselves—but if you intend to sleep with them in the trailer, you are out of your mind. Spend fifty dollars more and buy a tent, one that sleeps only two.

Hans Selye, the Wizard of Stress and Distress, says

that just resting isn't the answer. One does not recharge batteries lying in bed. Far from it. Bedrest too is a form of stress and further weakens the body housing the tired mind. The best way to grow strong and eager again, to build enthusiasm back to enjoyable and useful levels, is by doing something active *that you enjoy doing.* That's no problem for the people who were raised by active parents. The children of skiers usually ski and then teach their children the sport. Tennis players, golfers, and sailing enthusiasts present these useful antidotes to stress to their offspring at an early age, and campers have been known to backpack their babies as the first Americans did. But what if you were not so fortunate? What if there were no athletic models to copy, what if you really don't know how to begin? Then there are some very down-to-earth questions that must be asked, and the first one is: *What would I like to do if I had my druthers?* Then: *What are my limitations?* Limitations come in two parts, labeled *now* and *later.* For example, I'd love to ski in Davos next winter but (a) I don't know how to ski and (b) I can't afford it. Those are called *now* limitations. *Anyone* can learn to ski by first concentrating on building the strength and flexibility needed for the sport and *then taking lessons.* There are inexpensive ways to spend ski weekends, and books by the dozen will tell you how, once you have learned the sport. The *then* limitation, which is financial and applies to some time in the future, will be taken care of by time. One day you will either have enough put by for Davos, or you'll find places closer to home that will do almost as well. The constant, of course, is that either way you have learned to ski. The requirement for that was building the body needed for what you wanted to do *before* the season—*before* setting out on your vacation. That can be done successfully with nothing more than the *sexercises* in this book, and that goes for any sport you have in mind.

It should probably be brought to your attention that driving to wherever in your car, pub-crawling every night, sleeping until noon, shopping and sightseeing the rest of the day until it's finally time to start crawling again, may be lots of fun, fill your house with exotic bargains, and tote up an impressive list of famous places and fourteen boxes of slides—but it won't do a damn thing for your sex life. If you want to make the most of your vacation time and make every minute count, go into year-round training using every weekend as a mini-vacation and bits and pieces of your daily life as micro-vacations. And use that most deadly of our pleasures (far more dangerous than smoking, drinking, or over-eating), the television set, to help you set up what might be called mini-minute prevacation training programs.

Look over your daily life and find the areas where exercise could be instituted. For office workers there is the transportation to the bus, train, plant, or business. Instead of the car, *walk*. Instead of parking in the same building or out in the adjacent lot, get a spot blocks away and *walk*. Rather than eat downstairs in the cafeteria, find an eatery a mile away and *walk*. When you finish dinner, don't collapse in your chair, the good shows don't come on until later anyway, so after the news, call up a neighbor, grab your spouse or one of the kids, and go *walk*.

Stairs are one of the best pieces of built-in equipment you can find. Most stair risers are seven inches high. If there are fourteen steps to your flight, that's eight feet plus two inches per trip to the next floor. If your office is on the fifth floor and you make that climb twice a day, that would add up to eighty feet negotiated by your legs. Or put another way, 80 foot-pounds times your weight. If you weigh 175, you would lift 14,000 foot-pounds with your heart and lungs and 7,000 foot-pounds with each leg. At the end of each work week you could congratulate each leg on lifting 35,000 foot-pounds—or 1,720,000 a year, with two weeks off to really work them on vacation. But you can do even more than merely lift. By setting the ball of each foot on the stair and allowing the heels to drop down below the stair surface, you can stretch the soleus, or heel cords. Then, as you take the full weight on each foot, straighten the legs *and then rise to the toes.* By doing this you involve *all* the muscles in the feet in both strengthening and stretching exercises.

At home you can do even more with stairs. Turn on your record player, using a slow beat so you can work the whole foot. If you will do those fourteen steps thirteen times, you will climb a little over 104 feet and it will take a little over five minutes, or about two bands of popular music. Most mountain climbers require an hour to go one thousand feet; you will do a little better than that, and you don't need to do it all at once. Do that hundred feet twice every working day and you will have climbed Everest twice in a year without frostbite.

Mini-minute TV exercises are tied in with commercials and serve two functions. They provide exercise and they keep you too busy to trot out to the kitchen. When the commercial comes on, don't sit there staring like a zombie while some ad agency talks to you as though you were a moron. *Get up at once.* That's the key. *React immediately and every time,* and by the end of the week, your body will expect it.

First, do ten *waist twists* (exercise 8), counting one-chim-pan-zee, two-chim-pan-zees, etc., as you do them. Next, ten *bent over waist twists,* to the same count. That's twenty seconds gone. Then add five *snap and stretch* exercises (12) using one-chim-pan-zee for the snap back and the second chim-pan-zee for the stretch. Follow that with the *back stroke* (14), alternate for ten. Forty seconds are now gone. Finish with five *deep knee bends,* taking four seconds or chim-pan-zees for each one. That disposes of a one-minute commercial, relaxes your shoulders, rests and exercises back and torso muscles, stretches the chest, and improves your circulation.

For the second commercial you use your chair. Hold on to the arms as you face the seat, and standing on your left leg, bring your bent right knee to your chest. This strengthens the abdominals (and lessens the pot if you have one) as it stretches the back. Next, with the left leg held straight (your body bent over), kick your right leg back and up while keeping the foot straight (*not turned out*). Do ten with the right leg and then ten with the left. The kick back with the foot held in the straight position will strengthen your lower back and trim the hips. Follow this with ten *bent-knee kick backs* during which you *turn your foot out* on each kick. That works the sides of the hips which are said to sport lumps called "saddlebags." For the final twenty seconds, do the same five four-second *deep knee bends*. That disposes of the second commercial. The third minute should be dedicated to running in place, but wisely. Run in place for ten chim-pan-zees, using two steps per second, or running twenty steps. Run the next twenty steps with feet turned in and the next twenty with feet turned out. Half the minute will be gone, and if you are very out of shape, stop your running on that half-minute for a week, then add the other half with the following: ten apart-together jumps, twenty forward-and-back scissor jumps, and finish with twenty side-to-side jumps. By running in this way for a full minute, you will find that you work your legs and feet in a far more complete manner than you would by merely running in place with feet held straight or even running around the gym or the block. As the months pass, you may want to increase your running until you can use up two and then three commercials without stopping. This will greatly improve your endurance. In the course of a single evening you will get at least twenty minutes' worth of exercise even if you are stuck in a motel in a strange city, having left your gym shoes at home.

One of the most foolish approaches to a vacation is called *the last-minute approach*. The vacationers work up to the very last minute on Friday evening and then frantically pack bags, boxes, and the car right up to midnight. In order to get every single minute of vacation time, they start right off either before dawn or with its first rays and drive straight through, stopping only for meals and a snack. When they finally arrive, they are so exhausted that they hardly stir off the patio for the first week. By the middle of the second week they begin to feel like doing something active and fun, and suddenly it's time to pack the car and head back to the ghastly grind. Not only were they too worn out to do the things that might have renewed them, they were too tired to rest in a way that would have contributed to that all-important *growth and change.* They were probably too tired even to make love properly, and since they are still the same tired twosome who found it unexciting before they started out, they won't go home to much of anything either.

How, then, besides doing something active every weekend and using parts of every day to condition yourself, can you prepare for your vacation and really get the most for your efforts? First, accept the fact that your body is the only vehicle you will ever get in this life and that whatever you are able to put into your bank account will be totally useless if your health is allowed to deteriorate. Remind yourself too that if health goes, sexuality goes too, and that will end one of life's most delightful aspects. *No job is worth that.* If your work permits only two weeks' vacation, then at least two weeks are your right. Start slowing down a full week before you are scheduled to leave. You needn't feel guilty, you'll be twice as useful when you get back. Don't wait to get your gear together until V Day, do that the weekend before. Instead of driving straight through, check your map and find a place you can stop en route, and quit driving early in the day. Swim a little, maybe play some golf or tennis, walk a trail or rent a bike—*do* something. A vacation doesn't depend on a place, it depends on the vacationers.

People with a sports background don't need any help when it comes to using vacation time in the service of *growth and change,* but many people do. For example, what can you do with a beach? Look around you at the many beach baskers. They lie there under a blanket of sun lotion for the entire two weeks, gradually turning to a well-done cinnamon brown. They *look* great (unless they are fat, and then they just look well done). Those folks are not for real. They are like the man who wants to be a bullfighter but really doesn't want to fight the bull. After their two weeks' tanning is over they return to their home grounds and their friends say, "Wow! You look great." What they are basing that on is merely color, and color fades very fast. In a few weeks they will be as flabby as ever and fish-belly-white besides. If they had known how to *use* the pool or the beach, they would have gotten a great deal more than color from their vacation.

When people go on a vacation in the hills with hiking in mind, they can check their progress with a map, but on a beach it's more difficult. If on your first day out you walk all the way to the inlet over two miles of sand, the next day you won't be able to walk down to the corner with feet flat on the ground. So limit yourself to one mile on that first day, even if you've been walking a mile around the block every day at home. Anytime you use muscles differently, they set up a clamor—even if the only difference is caused by changing saddle horses. If you've worked up to four hours a day riding Ol' Buck with no stiffness or soreness, expect trouble if you have to ride those same four hours on Ol' Bronc while Ol' Buck goes to another rider.

It's easy to lay out a beach mile. Check your stride against the tape measure you should always have along to check your body's progress. If the stride is 24 inches, walk down the beach counting each step made with your right foot until you total 660, then turn around and walk back. Incidentally, if you make a heap of stones at that point, you will be surprised to find your 660 right-foot steps will fall short of the first day's mark when you walk it the following day. That's because muscles unused to making distance through sand have shortened with stiffness—not enough stiffness to really bother you, but enough to be charted. Continue on for another 660 steps the second day, which will take you down the beach a full mile. Make another cairn and return. That will double your exercise session. Be sure to keep up a good pace. You can set one for yourself with the use of the now-familiar chim-pan-zees. You will keep up a steady beat of 120 steps a minute if you say "one-chim" as you step on your right foot and "pan-zees" as you follow with the left. Count up to sixty chim-pan-zees and you will have used a minute, and one mile will take 22 minutes at that rate. While you are doing your brisk pacing, take a good look at the slow folk ambling along looking for seashells. Resolve *never* to let yourself fall into such disrepair—not at *any* age.

On the third day you will have two cairns to check against, each at the end of a half-mile, and you will find that your stride has lengthened again as the initial stiffness worked out. Carry on for another half-mile and return. By the fourth day, when you are walking four miles and your muscles are working like well-oiled machines, you will outdo yourself at each and every cairn—without conscious effort.

If jogging interests you, then remember that running in sand is not the same as running down the road or around the gym. Lay out your course of one mile just as you would for walking—*by walking*. Then jog the distance by running 25 steps (count only those made by the right foot) and walking 50. Alternate running with walking down to your half-mile cairn and back. *Then go swimming.* Your loose-ankle kick will relieve any tightness in your heel cords. As the days pass, you can combine the longer distance with an increase in your running steps, five a day. In five days you will be running 50 and walking 50 without paying for it by having to sit out a single dance in the evening. On the sixth day, start dropping the walking steps at the rate of ten a day. You will soon be running the full mile painlessly and almost effortlessly. Try to start off by running that full mile, and you'll have to join the beach baskers.

Water is a great conditioner, but most people use it

merely for cooling off from time to time as they deepen their tans. If you want to make the pool pay off on your vacation, buy fins, mask, and snorkel. If you have never used a mask and snorkel, put them on and wear them around the house a few minutes each day until you become used to them. Do that *before* you head for the cape. When you *and your subconscious* know that you won't suffocate while trying to breathe through the snorkel, run the tub full of water and toss in a handful of loose change. Get into the tub wearing them and put your face in the water. Breathe easily as you pick up the coins one by one. You will then believe (as will your subconsious) that the mask is watertight and you won't drown. Then, when you get to the pool, go into the shallow end, lie prone with your arms trailing, and kick your way across and back a few times. That slow step-by-step process can of course be cut considerably if you are a good swimmer already, and by taking it even more slowly, the person who has never been able to swim can learn how in record time.

Fins are a great asset in the water; you move much faster and cover greater distances, but they take more effort than swimming with naked feet. The resistance of the water to their much greater surfaces requires your leg muscles to put out considerable effort. Thus, if you swim a mile (there are 5,280 feet in a mile; check the length of the pool and determine the number of laps you will have to swim to achieve a mile, a half-mile, a quarter-mile, and your start, an eighth of a mile), you will do it faster with fins but with more effort. That means more and faster results from your training program.

The use of mask and snorkel protects your eyes from chemicals and salt, and they will let you see through water as though you were in your living room. That may not be worth much in the pool, but wait till you are proficient enough to try them in the sea, lake, or river. This is the way adventures begin; the tame little vacation spent at the shore while sharing a cottage with your in-laws can one day lead to a coral reef in the Caribbean.

The principles involved in having a happy worthwhile vacation, one that will relax both body and mind and help you to find the interesting elements within yourself, are simple:

1. Prepare your body ahead of time for whatever activity your vacation is to be built around.

2. Since your way of life is probably sedentary, make *most* of your vacation activities physical. (If your daily life *is* mostly physical, then you can feel freer to invest more of your vacation time driving the car or seeing the sights.)

3. Take care not to get yourself locked into schedules.

4. Use some of your time just for being and dreaming. Does that mean that you will never get to see the Louvre? Of course it doesn't. It means choose and plan wisely with both body and mind in mind. If you've always wanted to see Salzburg, Florence, or Dublin, by all means go right down to the travel bureau and pick up the literature. But while you are there, find out how far Salzburg is from the Dachstein and its trails. How you get from Florence to the Dolomites and where you rent your touring bike outside of Dublin. There's nothing that says you shouldn't sit in a canoe and fish in Canadian lakes, but you'd do better to sign up for a canoe trip that includes fishing *and paddling and portages.* San Francisco is a beautiful city, and you wouldn't want to miss it *on your way to a hiking trip in one of the National Parks.* Seeing the country from a car can't be compared with being a part of it on your two good legs.

5. And never forget what a vacation really is—a passport to yourself.

14

Conclusion

Someone, bored, weary, and wise, once said that the trouble with life is that it is so *daily*. Someone else, neither bored nor weary, but certainly experienced and perceptive, said that the only time life is worth living is when one is in love. Both statements apply to most of us. Life can become terribly repetitious, frustrating, and *daily*; it is also demanding, often limiting, and always unrelenting. If something doesn't happen to interrupt its pressures and demands, we are in danger of developing an attitude toward it that combines both fatalism and despair.

Whenever we love, however, all that changes. Six o'clock is no longer just the time when the alarm goes off, it becomes sunrise. People around us take on new virtues and dimensions, and best of all, we see new virtues and dimensions in ourselves and begin to guess at our own wonderful potential. We stop fretting at minor frustrations; indeed, we no longer notice most of them, so intent are we on the miracle within.

Being in love, then, is a highly desirable condition, and being loved follows as the next logical step. We should not overlook the fact that being loved often opens floodgates within us and makes it possible for us to love in return. The instant we are aware of love, we enter an inevitable cycle. Our bodies react with an increase in the flow of hormones, which in turn heightens awareness. This condition shows in our faces, the way we sit, stand, lie, even laugh. Others—not just the special person we love, but almost everyone—suddenly become aware of us, and we in turn are aware of their attention. We revel in it, catch it, toss it back, and use all of living as a sounding board for the secret within. If this has *ever* happened to you, you know it is true. If it has not yet happened to you, you are in for some beautiful surprises, but don't wait until you are attracted to someone before you prepare to attract. You might not be quite ready, and it would be a shame to miss even one opportunity. Life is just as unpredictable as it is daily, and there are no signs announcing the approach of love.

You might lose your chance. If another person is *not* attractive, *not* healthy, *not* vital, and *not* outgoing and pleasant, *you are not going to try to make contact with that person,* not even for the short while it might take to find out that there is more there than meets the eye. On the other hand, if someone *is* attractive, healthy, vital, pleasant, and open to you, you *are* going to reach out. If both of you are also physically ready for love—and that means possessed of a strong, healthy sexuality—the meeting may be incandescent.

The existence of strong, healthy sexuality and your awareness of its presence cannot be hidden. The subconscious knows all about it and projects it to those around us. Occasionally it is identified as "warmth" or "vibrancy," sometimes it is inadequately referred to as "sex appeal," but by any name at all it is a positive quality that can be developed. Begin by knowing it is within you, and then, by enhancing and developing your body, the casing for all that you are and will be, give yourself the chance to make daily living into daily adventure, delight, and happiness. Today is the day to begin.

Index

www.ingramcontent.com/pod-product-compliance
Lightning Source LLC
Chambersburg PA
CBHW060235290526
45789CB00001B/56
* 9 7 8 1 4 6 6 3 7 8 5 5 1 *